Getting Better

Getting Better

A Report on Health Care from the Salzburg Seminar

Edited by

Herbert P. Gleason

OG &H Oelgeschlager, Gunn & Hain, Publishers, Inc.
Cambridge, Massachusetts

International Standard Book Number: 0-89946-053-4

Library of Congress Catalog Card Number: 80-23486

Printed in the United States of America

Library of Congress Cataloging in Publication Data

Main entry under title:

Getting better

Includes bibliographical references and index.
1. Medical care — Congresses. 2. Medical policy — Congresses. 3. Medical care, Cost of — Congresses. I. Gleason, Herbert P.

RA2.H4 362.1 80-23486
ISBN 0-89946-053-4

This book was made possible by a generous grant from The Pew Charitable Trusts.

Contents

Introduction

The 190th session of the Salzburg Seminar, entitled "Health Care — Allocating Resources in Urban Societies," took place in May 1979. There were thirty-eight fellows and seven faculty members from seventeen nations. In lectures, seminars, and discussion groups, and at meals and in the evening, they examined the problems and successes of their national systems in coping with the escalation of health care costs.

The session, arranged by Herbert Gleason and Maurice Lazarus, was undertaken in the hope that experts from many countries could in the course of three weeks together identify common problems and agree on some solutions to the transnational dilemma of distributing resources that are apparently insufficient to meet everyone's health needs. The results exceeded our expectations: Much less time was required to describe national systems; generalizations came tumbling out; and the fellows spontaneously organized what they called "syndicates" to propound guiding principles in various areas of care.

The conclusions reached in the session at Salzburg have special value for the United States in this period of debate about national

Much of the material in this introduction appeared originally in the *New England Journal of Medicine* on September 27, 1979.

health insurance. European nations, eastern and western, have had long experience with the problems of health care financing, whether by health insurance or national health service. Despite divergent approaches, all have experienced escalating expenditures, with an ever larger share of their gross national product committed to health care — more if the national economy has been flourishing, less if it has been stagnant. Apparently, the amount of total resources allocated to health care depends more on the relative wealth of a nation than on its particular system of payment or organization.

If Sweden, whose government owns the hospitals and employs the physicians, cannot avoid spending an ever larger portion of its gross national product on health care, then piecemeal changes, such as consumer cost sharing, physician fee setting, or even centrally budgeted national health insurance, are unlikely to control expenditures in the United States. Only a modification of demand, coupled with limits on expenditure and incentives to economize, can begin to contain the explosion in health care costs.

Today every force favors escalating expenditure, particularly the unrealistic expectations of consumers and the pressures to spend money for increased technology. For the most part, consumers are insured privately or by the government and make little financial contribution of their own. Physicians who make the buyer's choices have no incentive to control costs. Indeed, they may increase them in an effort to minimize the risks of malpractice suits by electing a wide range of technologic procedures. Institutional providers are also disinclined to curb their costs, at least when a third-party payer will foot the bill.

Participants at the seminar agreed that further unlimited financing would simply increase costs without greatly extending care. Instead, they favored the following specific, incremental changes:

1. The general health of the population can be influenced most through the promotion of healthful life styles. Great strides, such as those made so far in this century with sanitation, nutrition, vaccines, and antibiotics, are not likely to be made again. Today major health improvement in a society must come from improved habits related to smoking, alcohol, diet, exercise, and curbing violence, most notably in connection with driving.
2. More emphasis must be placed on primary care, on teaching patients how to take care of themselves, and on providing primary clinics in the rural and urban areas that are now inadequately served. The key persons to discourage overuse of the

health care system are the primary physicians. If they and their associates are compensated in a way that accomplishes that objective, costs will be reduced.

3. The elderly will absorb a steadily increasing share of total expenditures for medical care. Services to the elderly should be directed toward keeping them functionally independent, thus minimizing institutional care of all types. The problems of isolation, depression, and inadvertent drug abuse are often neglected. Only if they are approached by a variety of people — including social workers, nurses, and homemakers in addition to physicians — will the needs of the elderly for independent living, companionship, and self-care be met.
4. Decisions concerning the allocation of scarce resources may better be made in terms of locally, rather than nationally, perceived needs. Many countries are beginning to enlist consumers in the running of health care institutions and to recognize their competence in allocating scarce resources. Toward this end, more encouragement should be given to health services research.
5. Much of the technologic development of recent years is costly, and its effectiveness has not in all cases been documented. Far more evaluation of new technology is needed before its dissemination.
6. Scarcity of resources to meet general, basic needs presents ethical issues, which, surprisingly, have not been widely acknowledged. It was agreed that the problems of attaining equity in the distribution of scarce resources must be articulated if rational choices are to be made within our limited knowledge of need, demand, and effectiveness.

The chapters that follow contain material presented by the faculty members at Salzburg, tempered and enhanced by the discussions that took place there. They reveal no society that has found a way to satisfy all the demands of its people for health care. But they suggest the radical notion that appropriate care may often cost less than what is today offered as the best.

Ernest Saward, who was chairman of the faculty at Salzburg, lays the foundation for understanding the escalation in health costs and the controversy over economizing. Robert Maxwell's stimulating overview of health systems concludes that incremental rather than sweeping changes are likely to produce improved access to care at lower cost. And Sissela Bok raises the ethical dilemma presented by our search for both equity and economy. And David Hamburg shows how we can begin to check wasteful and inappropriate applications of promising but untried technologies. He suggests that continued scientific research can find ways to extend more comfortable life and identify procedures which in fact are pointless if not indeed harmful.

Writing on disease prevention and health promotion, Sir George Godber sets forth the complexity of implementing programs in those areas. While he wonders if the prolongation of life that such programs may produce would not entail costs at least equal to the saving in care of the prematurely ill, he makes clear that the alleviation of suffering and expense should be dramatic and immediate. His chapter on care of the elderly particularizes that theme in an area of soaring demand and shows that less costly programs can indeed produce more well-being.

Turning to systemic reforms, Robert Maxwell describes some of the benefits that can be secured by regionalization of control mechanisms. Haim Doron, in his chapter on the organization of primary care in Israel, shows how a system so perfected as perhaps only Israel can install provides accessible, timely, and economical intervention to the entire population. Herbert Gleason then takes that theme a step further and argues that greater consumer control of the delivery system can lead to more appropriate responses to medical needs, greater public happiness and, therefore, better personal health. Maurice Lazarus suggests a mechanism for controlling hospital costs.

We conclude with the fellows' report of the deliberations of the syndicates that they organized. It continues to commend itself as an extraordinarily sensible concensus from seventeen countries on a problem of great international importance.

Chapter 1

International Escalation of Health Care Expenditures

Ernest W. Saward, M. D.

Health care expenditures in most developed countries have continued to increase more rapidly than the productivities of the economies on which they are based. Health care currently consumes between 6 and 10 percent of each respective economy's total productivity and is now seen as burdensome by most national governments. Monies spent for health care compete with, and at times preclude, movement toward other national goals or priorities. The fact that health care expenditures appear as significant societal burdens is a rather new facet of health care.

For the past twenty to thirty years, most nations have been vigorously planning and implementing an extension of their health services both quantitatively and qualitatively. While varying from nation to nation, there has been great success at extending the advantages of contemporary medicine to more and more of their populations. And while the method and organization of these services has varied greatly, each year the expenditures for those services have increased faster than the economic bases. These increases have, in some developed nations, been as much as 10 percent per annum. This, of course, has led each nation to adopt various controls and regulations of health care expenditure in an attempt to rationalize this growing sector of the economy. The fundamental purpose of the health session at Salzburg was to examine this process, to determine the state of the art, and to see what further methods might be employed in attempting to solve this complex problem.

The uniformity of the increase in health expenditure is at first perplexing, because it occurs regardless of the political nature of the economy, the background culture, the commonly expressed societal values, or the methods of financing or organizing health care. Inasmuch as the phenomenon is international and cross-cultural, it must be presumed to be founded on a transcending set of values.

An understanding, however superficial, of the historical development of medicine and its institutions is essential for an understanding of present health attitudes. Many precedents in medical care have long lineage. To illustrate, a diorite column from Babylonia, now housed in the Louvre Museum in Paris, was inscribed 3700 years ago with what is called the Code of Hammurabi. On it we can see that medical fees were differentiated for different procedures, with one scale for nobles and another for servants. This historic practice, the two class fee system, continues to this day, as evidenced in various social welfare payment systems. In some respects there was little progress in attitude for 3500 years.

Another tradition of long lineage affecting the medical care process emerged as an early Christian phenomenon. Jesus, according to the New Testament, did something apparently quite unusual in His contemporary society. He gave attention to poor outcasts of society. It was thought that caring for these, not necessarily curing them, would "gain grace" for those who so emulated the founder of their faith. This tradition prevailed into the twentieth century in many places and was often an excuse for the very low wages that were formerly paid for hospital work. A large part of the workers' compensation was in the opportunity to "gain grace." As workers turn from spiritual reward to monetary recompense in a materialistic society, hospitals have had to respond with sharply rising salaries.

Medical care a hundred years ago had a very limited knowledge base and, in the light of present knowledge, certainly could be regarded as having little effectiveness. Many years ago a Harvard professor remarked that not until 1900-1910 did medicine approach an effectiveness at which an individual patient, being attended for an episode of medical care, would have a fifty-fifty chance of being helped by the encounter. This, of course, was said about medical care from the standpoint of the curative function. Little is said in such an evaluation about the caring function of medical care, so apparently common in the past and so often ignored in the present great emphasis on technical process.

Hospitals in the nineteenth century largely continued their long traditions of existence within a religious context. Caring for the sick poor was a charitable function. The well to do had little or no recourse to hospital. They were cared for at home by doctors and servants. While varying from country to country, those hospitals that were not based in religion operated as a function of local government and were funded by local taxpayers. Some were formed of the British tradition as nonreligious voluntary charitable organizations. In all countries, the total expenditures were low when compared with the scale of the national economies. Medicine was largely practiced on a fee for service basis, in which the fees were adjusted by the physician to the patient's presumed ability to pay. Indeed, the fees might be very handsome for the care of elite members of society; on the other hand, care, if there was any at all, for the disadvantaged was either an act of charity or an opportunity for perfecting clinical skills.

Against this background of the ineffectiveness of medical care in general, the charitable nature of the hospital for the sick poor, and the low expenditures on the part of governments for health care, we must look in contrast at the current state of affairs.

Illness, intrinsically, is always a burden. The concern of society for the high expenditures for illness, which are also a burden, have now produced in all developed countries some form of health insurance or direct government-supported service. Thus, the cost of illness is largely taken from the individual and mutualized across the group or the whole society. It is also clear that, in the period when medical care lacked effectiveness in the curative sense, it made relatively little difference in outcome whether one did or did not receive professional ministration. At that time, attitudes toward illness and death were likely to be based in religious belief rather than in the process of medical care. Disease and disaster were accepted as fate; the doctor was not a significant factor in outcome.

We have only to look to an event early in this century — the influenza pandemic of 1918-1919, when twenty million lives were lost worldwide. There was indeed caring for these sick, but nothing specific to cure. Those deaths were accepted by the surviving families as fate, and there was little hostility or bitterness to physicians or the medical care process. Expectations of the power of medicine were very low.

But by the mid-twentieth century a profound change had taken place. With the introduction of the antimicrobial drugs and the conquest of the common infectious diseases that previously had so occupied the attention of hospitals and physicians a great metamorphosis occurred. True, scientific medicine had been developing steadily throughout the twentieth century with little public involvement or acknowledgement. But suddenly, the public imagination was captured by these "miracle drugs" for dreaded infectious diseases, and a new belief system was born — a system that based its faith and hope not on theology, but on technology.

Following a dramatic beginning in the mid-1930s, there has been a great outpouring of scientific effort and clinical research upon most of mankind's great afflictors. The present major ills in developed societies — heart disease, cancer, stroke, and mental illness — have by no means been as susceptible to rapid advances in their fundamental cure as were the infectious diseases. We are still struggling with them, with what have been called "halfway technologies." These technologies, which are not curative, simply ameliorate on a temporary basis. But it is as a result of many of these seemingly miraculous, albeit "halfway," technologies that the public has developed, and had reinforced, an abiding confidence in the process of medical care. If one can restart a stopped heart — indeed, if one can transplant a heart from one human being to another — the belief in the power of scientific medicine can be very great. And the expectations that flow from that power, or seeming power, can be equally great. Such miracles have come to be expected of medical care.

The public believes, often as an article of faith, in our advanced knowledge in scientific medicine. It is true that such knowledge has greatly expanded in this century, but a familiarity with the basic developments in the biological sciences reveals that we have only begun to elucidate the building blocks of knowledge that are essential for further progress in clinical medical care. One may say that early in the century we had a few islands of knowledge in a sea of ignorance. Today, we probably have a whole archipelago, but there is far more sea than there is solid land.

In spite of that sea of ignorance, the public imputes to medicine all the powers of contemporary science. Take, for instance, the changes that have occurred in the lifetime of most adults, and examine how very powerful they are. To travel at supersonic speeds to foreign lands, to view live television with close-up views of sports events thousands of kilometers away, to land a man on the moon and watch his activities — all certainly reinforce one's belief in a technology poorly understood by the individual. Biomedicine is equally complex and is an equally difficult process to grasp. And it is accepted with as little reflection as a telecast by satellite.

But the public is seldom propagandized with our deficit in knowledge. Rather, it is constantly bombarded with the accomplishment of the latest turn of investigation, experimentation, or performance. As a result, the public and their political representatives have a very great belief in, and expectations of, the power of scientific medicine and medical technology. This exaggerated belief in the power of scientific medicine and technology underlies, in all developed countries, the rising level of expectation of what can be done with that expertise and has led to the rising expenditures in health care.

Every age has its enthusiasms; one of the enthusiasms of this age is for medical care. Just as the civilization of ancient Egypt devoted very large shares of its productivity to the creation of pyramids to protect its rulers' immortality with a luxurious lifestyle, and just as medieval Europe devoted a great share of its productivity to the building of cathedrals in a promise for a life hereafter, so also all developed cultures today are willing to devote great expenditures to scientific medical care processes in the hope of gaining a longer and better life. This dominant belief in the power of medical care processes to extend life, to make it more free of suffering, is so prevalent that the public and governments have only begun to examine its validity. So far, the belief is so strong that an ever larger devotion of resources to medical care seems to be inevitable. This belief system transcends national differences and is the driving force underlying the escalation of health care expenditures.

Ritual plays a large reinforcing role in any belief system. The high technology in the medical process, conducted in sterile gown and mask, added to complex apparatus connected to the body with tubes and wire, makes a strong impact on patient and family alike. General anesthesia enhances the ritual in that it provides an escape from reality and return, but with a changed body. There are very few medical agnostics in the recovery room.

Epidemiologists have now repeatedly shown that it is not the rising and tremendous technical complexity in the medical process that has improved the health of populations; rather, they point to the general improvement in the living conditions, sanitary standards, education, employment, housing, and nutrition of the public as having a direct causal effect. Indeed, most of the improvements in health, including those in the infectious diseases, had begun in the nineteenth century and were well under way prior to the more recent scientific contributions of curative medicine.

There has also arisen in the past decade, chiefly in intellectual circles and in some degree also in political circles, a professed disenchantment with the technical medical care process and the dominant belief system. To some extent this dissent is based on a rational advocacy of improvement in lifestyle and encouragement of health-promoting habits. It is also based on constructive concepts of self-help in order to break the dependency on professionals. This last view alone would be a valuable contribution to tempering the belief system.

The ethic of our time requires that for each and every sick individual, medical care processes must be continued until their effect is proven to be zero or negative. For example, one never asks as one intubates the elderly alcoholic who has just had his chest crushed by an automobile whether it is individually useful or socially cost effective to start the emergency room respirator. One simply starts it. One starts it regardless of what the ensuing discomforts and expenditures may be, and both are well known to be very great for the management of this kind of patient. If there is any gain, no matter how marginal, compared to the size of the input, our current ethic demands that one make the input. More is better. Hence the congruence of the belief system in medical care and the current ethical assumptions about its delivery process are such that, when combined with the technological development of our times, they result in the inevitable escalation of health care costs, regardless of the culture, the political system, or the method of organization of health services.

Of course, throughout the developed nations there has been governmental reaction to this cost escalation. One of the clearest statements came from the Canadian minister of health, Marc Lalonde. His policy statement — pointing out that medical care does not necessarily produce better health with further increases of its costs, but that health is derived from lifestyle, environment, and the individual's biological background — has since been echoed throughout the halls of most governments of the world. In the five or six years since this report was widely circulated, many governments have strengthened their initiatives in environmental health and in health education.

The old adage about an ounce of prevention being worth a pound of cure has found new prominence in the field of preventive medicine. The new wistful hope relies on preventive medicine to cut back on curative medical spending. But many of the advocates of preventive medicine have yet to demonstrate their cost effectiveness when they specifically involve the medical care process for their execution. The preventive procedures that can be implemented without the cooperation of the medical profession or of the individual — such as supplying pure water, providing sanitary sewage disposal, and other basics — are the most cost effective. Those that can be achieved by healthful behavior on the part of the individual are also cost effective, but here the major problem is one of initial motivation and long-term compliance. Aside from immunization, only a very few such as hypertension control and pap smears are cost effective when they involve the medical care process.

Despite this, the political rhetoric of prevention at present asserts that if the public adopts a more health-promoting style of living, the expenditures on medical care will be reduced. In other words, political leaders are exhorting the public to change behavior so that societal resources may be allocated differently. The ancient Greek ideal of health-promoting behavior for an intrinsically more enjoyable life is less emphasized. It remains to be seen if the cost-effectiveness argument is a strong motivator of the public.

Changes in lifestyle encounter profound difficulties in their practical implementation. It is not just a matter of communicating health-promoting information; it is a matter of motivating a behavioral change. As a rule, a subset of the population will quickly adopt whatever is the fad of the day in presumed healthful behavior, from high fiber diets to jogging. The majority, however, is usually unmoved. The promoters of healthful behavior often ignore the fact that individuals have radically different behavioral priorities. The promise of good health at an advanced age is readily discountable by youth that may have, here and now, an immediate problem of social acceptance. Thus, some of the youth of our nations smoke and drink as part of their social evolution, although they are well informed of the possible eventual consequences.

Favorable environmental change may also encounter differences of opinion. Control of inflation and the ideal control of industrial pollution may be opposing societal values. To clean the environment of industrial pollutants costs more to industry, but perhaps not to society, than not to clean it. The products of industry will thus cost more to the public if environmental control is strict. Inflation is thus aggravated. It takes a long-term societal view to accept inflation now, as a tradeoff of possible future benefit to the public health. The pendulum of political priorities swings to and fro: there is no simplistic resolution of how to move simultaneously to inflation control and pollution control.

Unfortunately, however, with the exception of the immunization for certain infectious diseases, the whole process of prevention appears quite undramatic. In preventive medicine one deals with taking actions, often to be maintained for a lifetime, with only a distant and hypothetically favorable outcome. By contrast, curative medicine often has an immediate, measurable, and sometimes miraculous outcome. It is the public's perception of this difference that allocates resources in their present pattern to curative medicine.

Furthermore, much of the healthful preventive behavior is a statistical gain and not necessarily an individual one.

The emphasis in health promotion materials often exaggerates dangers from unhealthful activities. To be sure, the majority of lung cancer victims indeed are smokers. But the vast majority of smokers do not get lung cancer; the majority of the regular consumers of alcohol do not get hepatic cirrhosis. The example of the drinking, smoking Winston Churchill at an advanced age can offset a very great amount of health education propaganda. This is not stated to detract from the latter activity but to indicate that heavy emphasis on the danger of illness rather than the pleasure of health may do little to decrease the expenditure on curative medicine. Alas, we are all mortal!

In almost every nation today there is some variety of discord between the direct providers of health care (the professions, the hospitals, and other institutions) and governments (local or national) that are trying to manage the expenditures incurred by these providers. As the costs of health services continue to escalate, the viewpoints of the various factions become divergent and controversial. In this respect it is well to distinguish political rhetoric from political action. Depending upon the source of funding of health care, national and local governments may have different and opposing views. Political bodies are largely influenced by the belief system referred to above, but the resultant expenditures are usually compromised by budgetary necessity. In addition, local politicians, elected to safeguard and advance the causes of their constituencies, cannot politically afford to advocate lessening of the sophisticated health care services within their own areas. Thus, the task of restraint falls to central government officials, who at a distance are often forced to discern the priorities for health expenditures as opposed to other national goals and priorities.

On the other hand, the medical profession looks upon itself as improperly burdened by the politicization of the issues of health care. It often expresses itself in terms of defending the "quality" of health care. "Quality" often appears to mean total professional freedom to pursue its own views. We are reminded of Clemenceau's statement that "war is too important to leave to generals." When one-eleventh or one-twelfth of a national economy is spent on health care, the question how it should be spent will hardly be left to physicians.

Physicians see progressive regulation and resource constraint as being both insensitive and inconsistent over time. And rapid governmental reversals of policy, no matter how rationalized, are particularly disconcerting to the professions. For example, after having built up large health manpower resources in each country, we are now becoming concerned that these manpower resources are the very generators of the expenditures we are trying to control. And having devoted great resources to increase these health manpower supplies, national governments now find that they cannot afford the consequences. A similar phenomenon is seen with the supply of hospital beds. After several decades of capacity building to bring convenient access of health facility to all, governments now recognize that they cannot sustain the operating costs of the abundance.

Decisions can be made at a distant governmental level with regard to kinds of health manpower or numbers of hospital beds or similar policies. The reaction at the local level of any reduction is usually one of opposition. Rationalization is occurring, but occurring very slowly. The financial burden of detailed compliance with government regulation is itself increasingly heavy. In addition to the employment of health professionals, the need for the large involvement of lay administrators, accountants, lawyers, computer programmers, and clerks is obvious in the contemporary hospital, as hospital administrations attempt to comply with mandated informational requirements.

In summary, in this century we have come from a period of relative ineffectiveness in curative medicine, with low expectations, low expenditures for health care, and reliance on religious belief for the behavioral management of sickness and death, to a broad transcultural belief in and high expectation of the value of scientific medicine and the medical care process that results from it regardless of its cost. Despite epidemiological evidence to the contrary, the public, and often their elected representatives, believe that the medical care process is their chief pathway of attaining a long and healthy life.

Thus, each nation finds itself burdened by the expenditures so engendered. Belief in the "miracles" of medical care has gone so far that it is now felt that if there is an inadequate outcome, no matter how grave the illness, the fault lies with those conducting the medical care processes and not in the process itself. The faith is now in the process, not the performer.

Technologic development has so multiplied the possibilities in the medical care process that any serious reflection will soon show that if all the possible procedures were done for everyone in a society, the society would expend its entire wealth on this exercise alone. Hence the rationalization and control of these health expenditures, already beyond the point of productive return for the investment made, need serious consideration in all the different national methods of financing and organizing health care.

The health care session at Salzburg revealed that we have already moved a considerable distance along this path in our attempt to control and regulate health care. While the methods are different in different societies, as they inherently must be, the following chapters show that we have a commonality of purpose that will rise above national considerations not only for individual improvement but for the good of all. This may be accomplished in part by the pressure of finite resources, in part by political expediency, and in part by the sort of consistent and persistent advocacy of a rational use of health care resources that this book contains.

REFERENCES

Council of Wage and Price Stability. *The Complex Puzzle of Rising Health Care Costs: Can the Private Sector Fit It Together?* A Summary of Hearings Held in New York, Chicago, San Francisco, Philadelphia, Houston, and Miami; a Compendium of Labor-Management Innovations in Reducing Health Care Costs. 1976.

Knowles, John H. *Doing Better and Feeling Worse.* New York: W. W. Norton & Company, Inc., 1977.

McKeown, Thomas. *The Role of Medicine: Dream, Mirage, or Nemesis?* London: The Nuffield Provincial Hospitals Trust, 1976.

Mushkin, Selma J., et al. "Cost of Disease and Illness in the United States in the Year 2000." *Public Health Reports* 93 (1979): 495-588.

Saward, Ernest W., and Andrew A. Sorenson. "The Current Emphasis on Preventive Medicine." *Science* 200 (1978): 889-94.

Zubkoff, Michael; Ira E. Raskin; and Ruth S. Hanft. *Hospital Cost Containment: Selected Notes for Future Policy.* Prodist, New York: Milbank Memorial Fund, 1978.

Chapter 2

Health Systems: An Overview

Robert Maxwell

The study of health systems is threaded with paradox. For example, there are enormous differences between systems, stemming from differences in their historical, economic, political, and social contexts; yet there are equally marked similarities in the basic challenges faced within these contrasting systems. This is the first paradox examined in the present chapter. The second paradox is the preoccupation with health care expenditures — at times, apparently, to the near exclusion of concern about what value these expenditures buy. And the third paradox discussed here is the inclination to look to other health systems for panaceas (which almost certainly do not exist) while ignoring much that can be learned from comparison and discussion. From a review of these paradoxes arises the case for a more selective approach to reform, which leads into the substance of the rest of this book.

THE FIRST PARADOX: CONTRAST AND COMPARABILITY

Seventeen nations were represented at the health session at the Salzburg Seminar. Each one of their systems differs from every other — and not merely in detail. Substantial differences might be expected between, say, West Germany and Thailand, Greece and Finland, or Poland and the United States, because of differences in wealth and in political systems. One might not expect the marked differences that also exist between, say, Spain and Portugal, or among the Scandinavian countries, or within the Communist bloc.

Perhaps the best way to avoid total confusion, yet grasp something of the enormous variety of health systems, is to select half a dozen countries to illustrate patterns within the total spectrum. The half dozen selected here are Thailand, Italy, Poland, West Germany, the Netherlands, and Sweden.

Thailand, with a national per capita income of $380 in 1976, has little to spend on health care. Its limited health care resources are mainly concentrated in Bangkok, so that there is a mismatch between the distribution of these resources and of the population. Three-quarters of the country's doctors, but only a fifth of its total population, live in the cities. In the rural areas there are some 2000 doctors and 36 million people, to give a doctor-population ratio of 1 to 18,000. In the cities the ratio is one doctor to 1500 persons.[1] Bangkok has its major hospitals and private medical practitioners, many of them specialists. In the countryside, on the other hand, medical services scarcely exist, the gap being filled in part by "traditional" practitioners and herbalists. Perinatal and infant mortality are much higher for the country as a whole than for Bangkok.

Government seeks to regulate the system without taking it over, to assist the poorer half of the urban population in obtaining access to services, and to extend primary care into the rural areas. Most health care resources are not under direct government administration. The government is thus faced with problems of how (with very limited funds) to pay for any improvements in health care, how to provide incentives in the rural areas, and how (if at all) to intervene in the existing voluntary and private sectors in the cities.

Italy has in recent years been undertaking revolutionary changes in the organization and funding of its health service. Historically these services have been highly fragmented.[2] Most towns have had their own hospital for centuries, frequently with a religious foundation. Since 1968 these hospitals have almost all come directly under the administration of municipal government. Up to 1975, hospitals were funded chiefly on a per diem basis through compulsory public insurance, dominated by one major scheme (IMAM). Outside hospitals, medical care was mainly provided by private practitioners, who received fees from the insurance schemes and directly from patients.

In 1974, the central government enacted a regionalized National

Health Service, strongly influenced in concept by the British system. The regions are allocated budgets, based partly on past expenditure and partly on population. They in turn are responsible for allocating budgets to the public hospitals and for seeing that the hospitals keep within their budgets and provide value for money. Primary care is to be planned, coordinated, and controlled by local councils, funded through the regions. Various attempts are being made to bring pharmaceutical expenditures (which are high by international standards) under control. It remains to be seen if the changed system will make a major impact on Italy's long-standing health services problems of underfunded hospitals, lack of financial control, fragmentation, and imbalances in the distribution of resources (particularly between north and south).

Poland's health system, like those in all the Communist countries, is primarily state financed and run. There is, however, some private practice in urban areas, and there are also cooperative schemes organized on a mutal insurance basis. All physicians must work for seven hours a day in the state system. In addition, they can undertake private or cooperative practice. Fees for private practice are uncontrolled and raise the income of some physicians to a very high level. Hospital and specialist medical services are based on the towns.

Primary care is organized in the towns through polyclinics, with separate services for broad client groups such as children, and in the rural areas through small health centers, manned by a physician, a dentist, and a small number of nurses. Most people pay part of the cost of health care through part payment for drugs and frequently by direct payment to physicians. There is an uneven distribution of physicians between cities and rural areas and shortages in some specialties (e.g., anesthetics and rheumatology). As in many Western countries, there is concern both about access to services (long waiting times and, in remote areas, substantial journeys) and about "unnecessary" demands. The whole health care system is the responsibility of a central government ministry, working through regions and local units of administration.[3]

West Germany is the archetype of health systems based on government-regulated mutual insurance. Although Denmark can claim older cooperative insurance schemes, Bismarck laid the foundations for the first national system of social security in Germany between 1880 and 1890. Today virtually the whole German population is insured for all health services through some 1500 locally organized or occupation-related schemes. The insurance base is echoed in most other Western European health systems (apart from Sweden, Britain, and most recently, Portugal), even though there are substantial differences in execution. In Germany the separate schemes coordinate their activities through state and federal associations.

On the delivery side, virtually all ambulatory care is provided in Germany by private practitioners working outside hospitals. The state medical associations, which are publicly chartered bodies, have a measure of responsibility for ensuring that medical services are available where needed. The State Associations of Sickness Fund physicians negotiate contracts and total expenditures with the insurance organizations and are responsible for meeting the fees of their individual members within the contract sum. Hospital services are the responsibility of the *Länder* (provincial governments) working within very broad federal guidelines. Teaching hospitals are financed and administered separately from other hospitals and fall within the educational system. The contacts between hospitals and medical services outside hospitals are tenuous. Public health programs (such as inspection and immunization) are largely the responsibility of local government.

Until recently, the main concern in Germany has been the sustained development of services rather than cost containment and rationalization. However, there now is increasing concern about costs, and German health care expenditures are among the highest per capita in the world. The principal hope for controlling further increases lies with the employers and trade unions who are the dominant forces in the German sickness funds.[4]

The Netherlands, like Germany, finances health services primarily through a large number of locally organized sickness funds. Seventy percent of the population is covered by compulsory insurance, leaving the wealthiest 30 percent the option of voluntary insurance; and everyone is covered through government subsidy for catastrophic risks. In addition, most people carry additional private health insurance, even if they are covered by compulsory insurance.

The country's health services are remarkable for emphasis on community and nursing home care and for perpetuation of voluntary foundations. For example, the Cross associations have no close parallel elsewhere: They are voluntary in origin, continue to be strongly local in flavor despite public funding, and provide a variety of preventive and home care programs, especially maternity and child care. In psychiatry, the Netherlands also has extensive community programs, at least in the main urban areas. In contrast to Germany, where general practice is now weak, the Netherlands relies on general practice (with payment by capitation) for primary care. Specialists will normally be paid by the sickness funds only if the patient has been referred by a general practitioner. Possibly in the Netherlands the threshold for referral is lower than it need be, but standards of specialist and acute care seem in general to be high. All specialist physicians have a hospital affiliation: some are salaried, but most senior specialists are paid on a fee for service or fee per case basis. Fees for private patients are much higher than for sickness fund cases.

In recent years the Dutch Government has been concerned to encourage preventive activities, outpatient services, and nursing home care and to promote regional planning and coordination. The overall impression is of a strongly decentralized health system, even though the country is relatively small and government is unitary.[5] Public and professional satisfaction are high, and medical care is virtually free of charge at the time of use. The key issue is how, without sacrificing the great advantages of decentralization, control can be gained over health care expenditures, which have continued to rise exceptionally fast by international standards.

Sweden presents features that are less completely developed in many other countries. Except for some ambulatory care from private physicians, services are free or nearly free at the time of use, as in Germany and the Netherlands, but public insurance plays a relatively small part in Sweden. Hospital services are financed mainly from general taxation and are administered by the counties. Indeed, the county and municipal pattern of hospital provision has always been the dominant one in Sweden. Charitable foundations have played a much lesser part than in most of Western Europe, while the central government's role in health services has been less patently executive than in, say, Britain or the Communist countries.

The system is more dependent on hospitals than any other, with a high ratio of hospital beds to population (152 beds per 10,000 population in 1974). The pattern of hospital provision is tightly structured, with three interdependent levels — namely, local district hospitals, larger county general hospitals, and seven regional referral hospitals. The system is also weighted toward medical specialists, with few general practitioners except in rural areas, which are served by government-employed district medical officers. Only a small (10 to 15 percent) minority of physicians in Sweden are in private practice, and many of those few are elderly.

Most other physicians are state employees, either as district medical officers or on the staff of hospitals. Since 1970, state-employed physicians cannot do any private practice. In urban areas much ambulatory care, including primary care, is based on hospital outpatient departments. Care of the handicapped and chronic sick is well developed and tends, like acute medical care, to be institutional in emphasis. Nursing homes are often closely linked to district hospitals, and acute and chronic care are well coordinated. In all, Sweden's health care arrangements are elaborate, impressive, costly, and perhaps a little cumbersome in their dependence on specialist care and government-administered institutional provision.[6]

The addition of other countries would illustrate further variations in systems, and far more detail could be given about these six. Such a brief summary does, however, show something of the range of variation, including the special problems and imbalances of a developing country, the general approach taken in the Communist bloc, and some of the differences among three of the most advanced health care systems in the world (Germany, the Netherlands, and Sweden).

However, the similarities are ultimately more important than the differences. Historically, every system has evolved along a similar path from a partial, fragmented, unbalanced collection of institutions, based on charitable or municipal initiative in the main towns, toward a complex and sophisticated pattern of services for the whole population. As services have become more sophisticated, they have also become far more expensive. Collective insurance schemes and government funding have paid a steadily increasing part of the total cost. And governments have everywhere become far more involved in the administration of health services. Even where (as in the United States and Germany) they are reluctant to tamper with private enterprise, they cannot escape being concerned with the effectiveness, fairness, and cost of the whole health care system.

THE SECOND PARADOX: COST AND VALUE

The 1950s and 1960s were decades in which health care expenditures increased relentlessly throughout the developed world at a faster rate than national income.[7] The brunt of this increase fell on government rather than on the private sector.[8]

By the early 1970s it was clear that a clash must soon develop between bids for further improvements in health services and other competing claims for public finance. The downturn in world trade and the strain imposed by sharply higher oil prices hastened the clash.

In contrast with the previous decade, the international pattern of health care expenditures in the 1970s is not uniform. The rising trend has continued in some countries, with little more than a temporary pause. In others, health care expenditures have stabilized as a percentage of the gross national product. The United States and Canada illustrate the contrast: in 1970 they were spending 7.2 and 7.1 percent of GNP, respectively. By 1976 the differential had widened substantially, the U.S. figure having continued to rise to 8.7 percent, while the Canadian remained at 7.1 percent.

Where the rise in health care spending has been checked, the change has required determined action by government. Hospital expenditure in particular has been sharply curbed. Some governments have employed global budgeting for this purpose (for example, the United Kingdom and most of the Canadian provinces). Line item review, establishment controls, and prospective rate setting have also been used. And some form of regional planning is almost universal, in an attempt to restrict the rate of growth and the duplication of expensive equipment and programs.

Physicians' incomes are more difficult to control than hospital budgets, but here also a marked tightening has occurred. Governments are much concerned with the negotiation of physicians' fee levels. The rates thus set apply to reimbursement from public funds, and it may be open to physicians to charge patients more. (Contrast Quebec, where physicians may not do this unless they opt out of the public insurance scheme altogether, with Ontario, where it is common practice.) Some form of review of medical acts performed is also increasingly common, especially when physicians are self-employed, since physicians have substantial discretion over the work they undertake and can respond to a curb in fees by altering the volume and mix of their services.

Pharmaceutical pricing also has received close attention, and several countries have attempted to restrain "extravagant" prescribing patterns, generally (as in New Zealand and France) by restricting reimbursement to a limited range of drugs, chosen on grounds of effectiveness and price.

Since health services are manpower intensive (typically 70 percent of health care costs are wages and salaries, and in the developed world some 4 percent of the working population are employed in health services), manpower numbers and earnings are a crucial determinant of costs. After a rapid expansion of medical schools in the 1960s, many governments have come to recognize more clearly the expenditure implications of physician supply and have sharply curbed physician immigration. Manpower planning for the other health professions is just as important in human terms and arguably even more essential to the avoidance of key manpower shortages, but no other profession has the same discretionary influence on levels of health care spending as does the medical profession. Hence the central importance of physician supply and distribution.

Conversely, since physicians represent only some one in ten health services staff, their rates of pay have less direct impact on health care costs than do the salaries and wages of the larger occupational groups, particularly nurses, ancillary staff, and administrative and clerical staff. Governments have therefore become acutely sensitive to levels of pay awards for these groups. Greater sensitivity to the cost implications of these awards, however, goes no way toward discovering how to achieve settlements without in the process creating bitterness among groups of employees and damaging patients.

Predictably, several governments have recently attempted to reverse the historical trend toward increasing reliance on government funding. The attempt may have been to pass responsibility back to another level of government — from federal to provincial in Canada, from government to the social security system in Israel, or from compulsory to voluntary insurance in Australia. It may also be to increase the charges to users, as in France and to some extent in Britain. The various attempts spring from a common purpose — to stem the drain on public funds, check the rise in consumer demand and expectations, and lessen central government's embarrassingly exposed role as arbiter within the highly complex field of social programs.

Whatever the success of these many attempts to restrain the rate of growth of health care spending, the paradox is that far less attention has been paid to the more important question of value for money. In the developed world, health care expenditures now account for up to a tenth of total income (as measured by GNP) and a fifth (or even more) of government budgets. That governments are concerned to limit these expenditures is natural. But common sense dictates that arguing about the precise amount should matter less than what people want to obtain for their money, what they in fact receive, and if a different pattern of spending would be better. The debate cannot be conducted intelligently without the type of information that we would look for in our own personal affairs. That a class of spending constitutes a substantial portion of our income means little by itself. Yet the lack of intelligible information on the impact of particular health care expenditures is frightening, as is the general lack of informed debate on the subject.

THE THIRD PARADOX: PITFALLS AND STRENGTHS OF INTERNATIONAL COMPARISONS

In recent years the international comparison of health systems has ceased to be a minority taste and has become fashionable. This is entirely logical, since health care — or at least health care spending — is now a major public policy concern. To learn one must compare. Unfortunately, the tendency is to look for the wrong lessons.

To a British visitor to the United States, it soon seems that Americans concerned with health services are divided into two irreconcilable groups — a minority that views the National Health Service as appropriate for the United States and a majority that can perceive no good in it. Both views are false, but they illustrate the failure to learn from international comparisons. No system is for export as it stands. It is a product of the history and culture that have produced it and is not readily transferable to another cultural context. Moreover, the adoption of another system wholesale could only make sense if some other system had found the answers to the main problems of health care delivery. That is not the case. While many countries can show some impressive achievements, each displays some mixture of strengths and weaknesses. Indeed, despite the great differences among health systems, the similarities are even more striking than the contrasts, in terms of problems encountered and uncertainty about appropriate solutions.

The temptation, then, is either to imitate some other system slavishly, without understanding its limitations, or to see a weakness and immediately discredit it. The lessons that can be learned from international discussion and comparison are different. Our perception and understanding of the main issues can be sharpened by demonstrating their occurrence across systems and by illustrating the different forms they take. Thus, at Salzburg we shared not only our common concern about health care costs, but also exploration of questions of fairness and ethics; of balance between hospital and other services and between prevention, cure, and care; of the case for selectivity in the introduction of ever more expensive new technology; of the duty to care appropriately for rising numbers of the very old and the handicapped; of increasingly complex health manpower and industrial relation problems; and of the importance of seeking to assess the impact of health care activities upon need.

Moreover, we can learn from one another's experience, from

failures as well as from successes. Indeed, the usual result of a carefully considered policy initiative in the health field is neither total failure nor undiluted success, but the creation of a new situation calling for a further response. To take equity as an example, countries like Sweden, the Netherlands, and Britain can all show substantial success in reducing inequities of service utilization related to income.[9] Other inequities remain in each of these countries. In Sweden there is less access to service in the rural areas, and recruitment of district medical officers remains difficult despite longstanding efforts. The Netherlands shows great geographic disparity in the distribution of resources — the north and east of the country are much less well endowed, even in relation to their more scattered population — and there are very substantial variations of quality among institutions.

The United Kingdom has been conscious for some time of inequity toward neglected groups of people, particularly the long-term mentally ill, the mentally handicapped, and the elderly. The record of the last ten years shows some increase in standards for these groups and also how intractable the problems of change are. More recently the United Kingdom has been preoccupied with geographic inequities in the distribution of resources and is seeking to move toward fairer, population-based budget allocations. Most people accept this aim, but are rapidly becoming aware of the dangers of making sharp changes in resource allocation with insufficient consideration of, for example, threshold levels for major referral centers and of the impact of the changes on levels of care. The problems do not negate the overwhelming case for greater fairness within the nation. They do, however, underline the complexity of the matters we are dealing with in health systems and the high probability that reform is more difficult than it appears.

The theme runs throughout this book that change is best made incrementally in health systems, learning from each step and preparing for the next.[10] Perhaps that sounds timid, and there are no doubt cases where progress is not possible without bold and radical reform. But proponents of sweeping changes, such as the introduction of national health insurance in the United States, had better recognize their strict limitations. National health insurance may improve access to care for some of the population and reduce the financial impact of catastrophic illness. Tremendously important as that is, many health care problems would remain unresolved and others would be exacerbated, including cost. The same problems of health and health care occur in most health systems no matter how different. They are unlikely to be removed by massive systems changes. Instead, they call for a more precise and selective approach, which has led us into the themes explored in the chapters that follow.

NOTES

1. The imbalance between city and countryside, which is typical of many poorer countries, is not confined to the distribution of physicians. It applies equally to other qualified health services personnel. See, for example, N. R. E. Fendall, in *International Medical Care*, edited by J. Fry and W. A. J. Farndale (Oxford: Medical and Technical Publishing Co. Ltd., 1972), pp. 208-9. See also the many references to Thailand in John Bryant, *Health and the Developing World* (Ithaca and London: Cornell University Press, 1969). Approaches to tackling the problems of health care in poorer countries are described in K. Newell, ed., *Health by the People* (Geneva: WHO, 1975). The Tanzanian attempt to build community self-help in the rural areas is important; for the background see O. Gish, *Planning the Health Sector* (London: Croom Helm, 1975).
2. The background of health services in Italy up to 1975 is described in Alan Maynard, *Health Care in the European Community* (London: Croom Helm, 1975), ch. 7.
3. For a fuller account of health services in Poland see M. Kaser, *Health Care in the Soviet Union and Eastern Europe* (London: Croom Helm, 1976), ch. 7.
4. Uwe E. Reinhardt gives a clear, well-documented account of health services in Germany and useful comparisons with the United States, in *International Health Costs and Expenditures*, edited Teh-wei Hu (Washington, D.C.: Fogarty International Center, 1976), ch. 10. W. A. Glaser, *Health Insurance Bargaining* (New York: Gardner Press, 1978), describes excellently the insurance arrangements in Germany. (The book also contains chapters on the Netherlands and Sweden.)
5. There are many short accounts in English of health services in the Netherlands, including, for example, J. G. Simanis, *National Health Systems in Eight Countries* (Washington, D.C.: DHEW, 1975); Glaser, ch. 5; and Maynard, ch. 3. *The Compendium of Health Statistics of the Netherlands*, published in English by the Ministry of Public Health and Environmental Hygiene, gives extensive factual information, but there is as yet no adequate English analysis of the complicated pattern of provision, with its emphasis on decentralization and its wide range of community services.
6. For a compact description of Sweden, see Simanis. For a more discursive analysis see Odin Anderson, *Health Care: Can There be Equity?* (New York: John Wiley & Sons, 1972), which compares the United States, Sweden, and Britain and concludes with the hope that the United States will move toward a Swedish rather than a British pattern. A more factual description of the organization of health services in Sweden can be found in Vicente Navarro, *National and Regional Health Planning in Sweden* (Washington, D.C.: Fogarty International Center, 1974); or in A. Lindgren's chapter in *Health Service Prospects* (Lancet and Nuffield, 1973). For background see also D. Wilson, *The Welfare State in Sweden* (Heineman, 1979).

7. See B. Abel-Smith, *An International Study of Health Expenditure* (WHO, 1967).
8. See OECD, *Public Expenditure on Health* (July 1977).
9. For a comparison of access to services in the United States and Sweden, see R. Andersen, B. Smedby, and O. W. Anderson, *Medical Care in Sweden and the United States* (Chicago: Center for Health Administration Studies of the University of Chicago, 1970). The study suggests that differences in income have less effect on differential access to services in Sweden than in the United States. However, there are residual class differences in utilization even in Sweden, as there also are in Britain. Achieving fairness for the disadvantaged is more complicated than merely removing financial barriers.
10. In the U.S. context, the classic statement of the case for an incremental approach to reform is by Eli Ginzberg in *The Limits of Health Reform: The Search for Realism* (1977).

Chapter 3

The Relevance of Moral Philosophy to Medicine

Sissela Bok

One of the simplest definitions of ethics — or moral philosophy — is that attributed to Epicurus: "Ethics deals with things to be sought and things to be avoided, with ways of life and with the goal of life."[1] Ethics, according to this view — and it is one I share — concerns human choice — individual and collective choice about the conduct of lives, goals and standards, and levels of integrity and concern to set for oneself and work out with others.

At issue in medicine are precisely such choices, insofar as they affect illness and health, life and death. All questions of moral choice that beset human beings can come up in medicine — and often do so with a special urgency and intensity.

Medicine is, in this sense, a magnifying mirror held up to human interaction in all its complexity. It magnifies because the encounters that center around illness reveal us all at our most vulnerable and touch on our most powerful emotions. When we are helped or injured by medical care, dealt with fairly or exploited, treated as autonomous agents or coerced, lied to or told the truth, this simply matters more to us than when we are dealt with in similar ways at less vulnerable times.

I draw, in this chapter, on my article "The Tools of Bioethics," in *Ethics in Medicine*, edited by Stanley J. Reiser et al. (Cambridge, Mass.: MIT Press, 1977).

It is not surprising, therefore, that of all the professions, medicine has the longest, most articulate tradition of applied ethical inquiry — a tradition carried on by great thinkers who were also physicians (Hippocrates, Avicenna, and Maimonides among them) and expressed through the centuries in medical codes of ethics, in oaths sworn by physicians, and in analyses of both general ethical problems and particular quandaries. How to help patients and, above all, not to hurt them; whether to treat all who ask for help or to turn away the poor, those of an enemy nation, or of an alien race or religion; how far to go in keeping confidential the secrets learned about patients; and what constitutes violation of a patient's modesty or physical integrity — such questions have been probed with remarkable persistence.

But these writings have not been unanimous — especially not on matters having to do with equality and with the distribution of scarce medical resources. True, some oaths in antiquity were eloquent on the subject. An inscription on the Sanctuary of Aesculapius, for instance, on the south slope of the Acropolis, reads: "[The physician] would be like God: saviour equally of slave, of paupers, or rich men, of princes, and to all a brother."[2] And a Canon of Medicine, China, Han Dynasty, 200 B.C.-200 A.D., holds that a doctor should

> pledge himself to relieve suffering among all classes. Aristocrat or commoner, poor or rich, aged or young, beautiful or ugly, enemy or friend, native or foreigner, and educated or uneducated, all are to be treated equally. He should look upon the misery of the patient as if it were his own .... One who follows this principle is a great doctor, otherwise, he is a great thief.[3]

Similarly, the oath long thought to have been written by Maimonides states: "Preserve the strength of my body and of my soul that they ever be ready to cheerfully help and support rich and poor, good and bad, enemy as well as friend. In the sufferer let me see only the human being."[4]

On the other hand, a Hindu oath reflecting a long oral tradition, prescribes as follows:

> No persons, who are hated by the king or who are haters of the king or who are hated by the public or who are haters of the public, shall receive treatment. Similarly, those who are extremely abnormal, wicked, and of miserable character and conduct, those who have not vindicated their honour, those who are on the point of death, and similarly women who are unattended by their husbands or guardians shall not receive treatment.[5]

By comparison, the absence of any thought that the physician should care equally for all is very striking in the Hippocratic Oath,[6] the most widely disseminated oath even today. Nor do the Principles of Ethics of the American Medical Association venture such a notion. Equal treatment of the sick has been asserted only sporadically and is absent in today's most commonly used codes in the United States.

The vaster questions of social justice have not, on the whole, been discussed at all in the historical documents. In the past, as now, principles of medical ethics have been primarily principles for individual behavior — between health professionals and patients or between one health professional and another. The increased pressure to consider moral principles governing institutions and societies is beginning to force attention toward questions of medical justice. What is a just allocation of medical resources — among citizens of a community, a state, or even the world? And what roles do equality, benefit, and avoidance of harm play in such schemes of allocation? These most important of all ethical inquiries are not addressed at all in traditional codes of medical ethics.

Incomplete and conflicting as they are, the traditions of medical thinking about how best to distribute scarce medical resources could nevertheless serve to shed light on many underlying moral conflicts. That this does not happen more consistently is due to yet another limitation: practicing health professionals and administrators often have but rudimentary knowledge of the tradition of ethical inquiry in medicine. They often fail to discern the existence of the moral choices that confront them each day. They may even be told — on hospital wards or in laboratories — that there are no ethical problems in medical practice, only good medicine and bad medicine. Even those who struggle to work out moral quandaries have few tools at their disposal. Meanwhile the public is increasingly concerned to have a voice on such issues as the distribution of medical care or the rights of patients. It will never again be possible to think of medical ethics as a matter for the health professions alone.

The questions of equality cannot be avoided if we are to address the ethics of distributing scarce resources. Should equality of access to medical care be the norm and the burden of proof fall to those who would give unequal access? And if inequalities are to be tolerated, what should be the criteria for distribution? Should need alone dictate the allocation? Or should factors like the ability to pay, or social status, or merit, or place of domicile also play a role?[7] Finally, what limits are appropriate to mark off the population that is to share the scarce resources?

ALLOCATION AND NEED

Consider first the criterion of need. Nowhere is it more difficult to apply than to medical care. In many aspects of life, human beings have quite similar basic needs — as for food, shelter, breathable air, drinkable water, and defense from assault. But the basic needs for medical care vary dramatically from one case to the other. Some go through life with little need for such care; others could use nearly limitless resources.

Add to this disparity the fact that the needs for a person's good health or recovery may go beyond that person, and extend to his family, to those to whom he might give the disease if not treated — even to the entire society, as in wartime.

For these reasons, rationing health resources is entirely different from rationing, for instance, water or gasoline. Yet these distinctions are not always made when a health resource has to be rationed.

Thus Henry W. Beecher has noted that the allocation of new substances such as insulin and penicillin when they are first coming into use and still very scarce is often ad hoc.[8] Insulin, in the early days of clinical use, was first given to individuals in desperate need, especially diabetic children whose mortality would otherwise be 100 percent. Among the candidates for assistance, one other criterion was used in the selection — psychological stamina. But when penicillin was first shipped to North Africa in 1943, it was not allocated to those whose need was most desperate; it went, instead, first to soldiers who had gonorrhea and who, with its help, could be returned to the battle lines in one week. Beecher concluded that allocation of scarce medical resources has often been based on intuitive — and at times conflicting — views of what is most fair or most beneficial.

Another difficulty confronted by those who would allocate scarce health resources according to need is that the effort to satisfy one need in a fair and equitable manner may give rise to new disparities with respect to other needs. Health needs may come to be given a new priority as compared to the needs for education or for economic assistance to the poor. Or else health care assistance given according to acuteness of need may be disproportionately allocated to persons in one age group, to the detriment of others. Or the resources may be partially exhausted in caring for the present generation, to the detriment of future ones.

Yet another way in which disparities may arise through the very effort to distribute fairly is illustrated by the early allocation of kidneys to transplant and of kidney dialysis in the United States. Confronted at first with extremely limited resources and a great many applicants for assistance, hospitals in the United States worked out criteria in addition to that of need — absence of hypertension, for example, or a physiological age of seventeen to fifty years, financial resources, and at times, "value to the community." The patients who were rejected died — perhaps for having too little money, or because of having been judged uncooperative, or even because of being a prostitute and thus judged less valuable than other patients.[9]

In part because of the troublesome nature of using such criteria for selection, the U.S. Congress passed legislation in 1972 requiring government payment for almost all patients on artificial kidneys or who needed a kidney transplanted.

As a result, patients in need of this kind of assistance are now on a much more equal footing from the point of view of access; but the costs are so high ($1 billion at the end of 1977, $3 billion estimated for 1984) that those who suffer from other diseases and need similarly expensive assistance are now less equitably treated, in terms of access to health care, than before.

This example points out, in addition, yet another set of difficulties with respect to the equitable distribution of scarce resources: What should be done if an allocation is made that turns out to skyrocket, singling out a group of recipients for resources that cannot be granted all who suffer as much? What are the ethical considerations in stopping ongoing support to existing identifiable individuals — on dialysis, for instance? How is stopping something different from never having begun it in the first place?

RANGE OF DISTRIBUTION

Underlying these difficult questions of allocation is an even more fundamental one — that of the range of beings to whom some form of medical care might be not merely helpful but actually owed. The current debates about what is owed to the human fetus, to animal subjects of research, to persons in permanent coma, or to the very old center around this issue.

These debates in medicine reflect a central tension within philosophy as well: Toward whom might some moral consideration be due, at least in principle? Who counts as a legitimate possessor of rights?

Health care resources are at present disproportionately allocated among different nations. The fairness of such a distribution is under increasing debate, as is the way in which the allocation is influenced by trade and aid policies from without and by corruption and maldistribution within so many countries.

Even within a nation, the question of who is to count as a participant in schemes of allocation underlies a great many conflicts. In medicine as in philosophy, universalists have battled against holders of parochial views of kin or clan, class or race. Those who argue for a universal range usually take it to be identical with the category of human beings. The distinction between the human and the nonhuman has often seemed relatively unproblematic to its holders when compared with the battles to ensure that all human beings be entitled to certain equal rights.[10]

In order to avoid or supplement a religious justification for the human-nonhuman dividing line, some quality is usually put forth as underlying the respect due only to human beings. Many — among them St. Augustine and Kant — use the Christian distinction between those who possess reason and all other beings.[11] And John Rawls claims that which distinguishes those who are entitled to equal justice is a "capacity for moral personality" — "those who can give justice are owed justice."[12]

Such criteria — reason and the capacity for moral personality — call forth the very natural objection that some humans — among them the immature, the unconscious, and the injured — do not, or do not yet, possess these characteristics, yet are nevertheless thought to possess rights. (Contract theory, in particular, has difficulty here: it has to stipulate some significant reciprocity between those of whom justice is asked and those to whom it is owed; yet most of us do not in fact regard those two categories as coextensive or reciprocal.)

The traditional answer to this objection is to say that we must include in the protected category not only those who actually exhibit the particular quality, but also all who have potential for it. In this way, children and those whose capacity to reason or to act morally is temporarily injured or in abeyance can be included.

Yet potentiality raises immense difficulties, as well as opportunities for error and bias — how to decide when potentiality is present; what likelihood or minute chance of potentiality is to count; whether the burden of proof rests on those who want to exclude or to include borderline types of potentiality; and who is to decide in case of conflict. Medicine shows up these difficulties in concrete detail, as in the Karen Quinlan case. Should obligations to her depend on the fraction of a fraction of possible partial recovery that could not be ruled out?

In the Karen Quinlan case, the difficulty stemmed in part from the uncertain prognosis. But other medical cases illuminate still more perplexing difficulties in determining the range we should grant to moral obligations. First of all, what do we owe to those who, while genetically human, are not ever going to possess the capacity to do justice or to reason — the baby born without a brain, for example, or persons who, unlike Karen Quinlan, are quite certainly never going to be able to breathe without machines, sunk in deep coma with no end in sight? Can they be allowed to expire? Used for experiments too risky to be performed on others? Killed?

Second, what do we owe to those who may not even be human, but who possess attributes of rationality and who are very clearly capable of suffering from our acts? Is it right, for example, to cage female chimpanzees and to impregnate them again and again only to experiment on them with different methods of abortion? And what of the hypothetical beings with part human and part nonhuman genetic material? Or animals with greater intelligence than many humans?

Third, what do we owe to those beings who have not yet developed even rudimentary personhood — the newly formed embryo or human beings not even conceived? We can now predict how likely it is that a couple will, if they conceive, have a child with any one of a number of illnesses. If a man and a woman know that any baby they conceive has a 50 percent likelihood of having hemophilia and that society will have to use increasingly scarce and expensive resources to deal with this affliction, can they regard their unborn child as having a right to this medical care? And do they themselves have an unlimited "right to procreation" no matter how catastrophic the predicament they might impose on their children and on society?

Who, among all these beings, qualifies for belonging to the "others" whom the Golden Rule enjoins us to treat as we would ourselves be treated? How would a principle of equality or one of doing no harm apply to them? The traditional views of humanity and rationality and moral capacity falter in such circumstances; not one of them is either necessary or sufficient as a criterion.

The capacity to suffer is sometimes brought forth as an alternative criterion and as a way of declaring the human-nonhuman distinction illegitimate. This criterion is no more capable of being used on its own than the earlier ones we have mentioned. It can be used only as a corrective for the others. So used, it can help us, for instance, to avoid the absurd predicament of advocating the preservation of genetically human cells at all costs — even in the earliest hours of pregnancy or when a spontaneous abortion of a severely malformed fetus is taking place.

The capacity to suffer as a partial criterion corresponds, moreover, to our sense that the nonrational, the nonmoral, the beings not longing for what is beyond this world can in fact be wronged. The fact that they can be hurt and can suffer through our actions seems closer to giving a good reason to weigh the morality of what we do to them than the fact that they possess some genetic, moral, or intellectual potential.

Health care and research should help us to rethink these categories and dividing lines — to rethink them in contexts of illness and health, life and death. Many societies have gone about allocating health care resources haphazardly and without confronting the underlying ethical questions. They have allocated at times with bias, often with a lack of foresight; they have dislocated fragile structures, created unnecessary dependencies, brought about new disparities, backed into sudden reversals. They have done so in part out of a failure to see the ethical issues at stake.

The need is great to think through these questions and to debate them with respect to both collective and individual choice. Doing so would be no guarantee that choice would improve; but it is hard to see how one can approach such choice without articulating the ethical issues and debating them as rigorously as possible.

In the United States, the last decade has seen an unprecedented growth of interest in ethical questions, both in public debates and in the education of health professionals — a movement reflected, in turn, in a great many other professions as well. By now, almost half of the country's medical schools have instituted serious courses in medical ethics. The ethics of nursing and of the allied health professions is finding room in more and more courses. An articulate literature has sprung up, with journals and textbooks of high quality.

These developments are a response to the urgency of the conflicts confronting our institutions with respect to providing health care. As Mary Midgley points out, philosophy — and therefore ethics — "like speaking prose, is something we have to do all our lives, well or badly, whether we notice it or not. What usually forces us to notice it is conflict."[13]

NOTES

1. Diogenes Laertius, *Lives of Eminent Philosophers,* X.30.
2. M. B. Etziony, *The Physician's Creed* (Springfield, Ill.: Charles C. Thomas, 1973), p. 21.
3. Ibid., p. 20.
4. Now attributed to Marcus Herz and thought to have been published in 1783. See Etziony, *The Physician's Creed,* pp. 29-31.
5. Ibid., p. 15.

6. The Hippocratic Oath makes use of equality only in the limited sense that the physician foreswears sexual advances to those in the household of the sick, be they female or male, free or slave.
7. See Gene Outka, "Social Justice and Equal Access to Health Care," in Tom L. Beauchamps and Le Roy Walters, eds., *Contemporary Issues in Bioethics* (Encino, Calif., and Belmont, Calif.: Dickenson Publishing Company, 1978).
8. Henry W. Beecher, "Scarce Resources and Medical Advancement," *Daedalus* (1969): 275-309.
9. See Renée Fox and Judith Swazey, *The Courage to Fail: A Social View of Organ Transplants and Dialysis*, 2nd ed. (Chicago: The University of Chicago Press, 1978).
10. See Peter Singer, *Animal Liberation* (New York: Avon Books, 1975) for a challenge to this view and for a history of past challenges.
11. St. Augustine, for example, holds, in *The City of God Against the Pagans* (Cambridge, Mass.: Harvard University Press, 1957), Book I, Ch. XX, that men can kill animals and plants, since these latter have no reason, and that "by the altogether righteous ordinance of the Creator both their life and death are a matter subordinate to our needs."
12. John Rawls, *A Theory of Justice* (Cambridge, Mass.: Harvard University Press, 1971), pp. 504-12.
13. Mary Midgley, *Beast and Man: The Roots of Human Nature* (Hassocks, Sussex: The Harvester Press, 1978), p. xiv.

Chapter 4

More Judicious Use of Biomedical Technology

David A. Hamburg, M.D.

Medical technology has advanced at a prodigious rate in the past twenty years, changing and improving our ability to prevent, detect, and treat disease while raising still higher the public's expectations about medical care. Hundreds of new technologies enter the health system each year, and there is no reason to believe the pace of change will slacken in the foreseeable future; if anything, it is likely to increase.

The benefits of new technology have frequently been clear and convincing. Examples abound of new equipment and procedures that have significantly advanced the practice of medicine, from CT (computed tomographic) scanners for use in early detection of brain tumors to a variety of new surgical procedures useful in treating heart disease. Some new technology has reduced the cost of providing health care, some has increased access to care, and some has improved the outcome of care.

The blessings have not been unmixed, however. New equipment, procedures, or systems often come into wide use rapidly, before they

I wish to express my deep gratitude to Martha Angle for help in the preparation of this paper and to many colleagues in the Institute of Medicine who have participated in its work on this subject.

have been subjected to well-designed research on their relative effectiveness.[1] Many involve significant risks, some intrinsic and some that vary according to the setting and skill with which they are applied. Much of the new technology is increasing the cost of health care, sometimes dramatically.[2] At a time of economic strain and intense public concern over inflation, expensive machines and the expensive experts who employ them are coming under sharp and sometimes hostile scrutiny. Unless we are fostering this "industry" as an economic stimulus per se, we need to develop better methods for distinguishing useful from nonuseful interventions, keeping an attentive eye on the ultimate objective — improved health for individuals and populations.[3]

Medical technology can be broadly defined as any kind of knowledge or skill intended to improve health. More precisely, it is the "techniques, drugs, equipment, procedures — and systems combining these elements — used in the delivery of medical care."[4]

The development of biomedical technology (as distinct from its diffusion) involves creative activities that culminate in new technical capabilities. It requires a dynamic interplay of clinical, biomedical, and engineering talent in proportions that vary according to the particular application intended. Development can take place in a variety of settings. Surgical technologies, for example, are often developed in an academic medical center, while a new drug is most likely to be produced in an industry laboratory. We have much to learn about the conditions that foster clinically valuable innovations.

In principle, new technology should be introduced into the practice of health care (i.e., diffused) when its benefits to society outweigh its costs. In practice, however, knowledge of either benefits or costs is often very limited at the time decisions regarding the dissemination of a new technology are first made. Current methods for evaluating new biomedical technology are neither timely nor coordinated, and usually they do not consider economic implications.[5]

In general, technology used in hospital (and clinical) services is subject to strong pressures for adoption and tends to spread quite rapidly — usually without concomitant research to clarify the advantages and limitations of different uses, and with little or no analysis of cost. Indeed, prevailing methods of reimbursement by public and private third-party payers encourage increased provision of technology-intensive services, even without strong evidence to show commensurate benefit to the patient.

Motivations to use technology-intensive interventions include a desire to improve health, directly or indirectly; a desire to participate visibly in a technology-oriented society; increased earnings for practitioners and manufacturers; and the expectations and demands of patients, who have been conditioned by the mass media to invest great faith and hope in technology of all types. Taken together, such factors, operating both consciously and unconsciously, provide a powerful set of incentives for the use (and overuse) of technology in health care. At the extreme, technology becomes a new kind of magic, reinforced by the powerful and pervasive wish for good health that characterizes so much of human behavior.

The health professions intend to be — and the public expects them to be — science-based. This implies the extension of scientific methods and evaluations to the entire care system insofar as feasible if we are to assure the quality of health care in terms of known efficacy, safety, and cost effectiveness. Yet scientific assessment of medical technology and its uses is extremely limited at present.

New drugs are the only type of biomedical technology currently receiving adequate research scrutiny, but even this evaluation is significantly limited in the United States, since it is conducted prior to marketing and there is very little monitoring once a drug is approved and released for general use. The Food and Drug Administration, which evaluates new drugs, also conducts limited assessments of medical devices, but such testing is sharply restricted to certain aspects of technical validity. Once we leave drugs and equipment, scientific assessment becomes the exception rather than the rule. Carefully derived recent estimates indicate that only 10 to 20 percent of all procedures currently used in medical practice have been shown to be efficacious by controlled trials.[6] Clearly, major improvements are needed in our information base and in the processes used in generating it. This is not surprising in view of the very recent emergence of modern, science-based medicine and the very rapid changes of the past decade.

The central challenge facing us is to create or strengthen processes that both foster innovation and provide a timely scientific assessment of new biomedical technology. Such assessment can help (1) insure that technologies are made available when they are shown to have probable benefits with acceptable risks, (2) constrain the diffusion and use of technologies that either lack efficacy or cause excessive harm, and (3) provide evidence to guide appropriate use of all technologies, new and old.[7]

It is important, when assessing efficacy and safety, to recognize that results may be quite different in average use conditions, such as a community hospital or physician's office, from those obtained in carefully controlled research conducted in the highly favorable setting of an academic health center. Therefore, assessments of a particular technology under near-optimal conditions represent only the starting point — albeit a crucial one — in the effort to evaluate its potential benefits and risks. Such assessments, if positive, should then lead the way to tests in community settings more characteristic of the circumstances in which most patients receive their care.

All research must have a "market" — individuals, institutions, or organizations ready to use the information in making decisions. In the case of research on medical technologies, this market includes patients, physicians, hospitals, third-party payers, and public funding or regulatory agencies. Different criteria can be used to evaluate a particular technology, depending on the objectives and interests of those seeking the information. Physicians, for instance, will be more interested in information about efficacy, safety, and appropriate use guidelines than they will be in data about anticipated costs. Third-party payers on the other hand, will be acutely concerned about economic considerations.

An Urban Institute Conference on Medical Technology sponsored by the National Center for Health Services Research in December 1978 considered five general evaluative criteria that can be applied in varying circumstances.[8]

1. Technical validity — the extent to which a medical technology does what it purports to do and does it safely.
2. Effectiveness — the extent to which a technology achieves a specified health objective.
3. Cost effectiveness — the extent to which a new technology represents the least costly way to achieve a specified health objective.
4. Net social benefit — the extent to which a technology is worth its costs (a value judgment).
5. Societal impact — the effect of the technology on the social, legal, and economic structure of society.

Each criterion is relevant to certain types of decisions, each builds on information developed in studies designed to answer preceding criteria, and the appropriateness of each depends on the maturity of the technology as well as the needs of the decisionmakers.[9]

Regardless of which criteria are applied in evaluating a particular technology, there remain the questions of how to strengthen the processes of research on technology in health care and what to do with the information generated. In essence, a logical sequence for this purpose would include the following basic elements:

1. Identification of technologies that need evaluating.

2. Testing through application of some or all of the criteria stated above.
3. Synthesis of the information gathered, which may well include interpretation of the evidence and judgments or recommendations about appropriate use.
4. Dissemination of the synthesized information to interested parties, including health professionals, manufacturers, reimbursement agencies, and the public.

Any attempt to evaluate new medical technology and reach some judgments about its usefulness will inevitably be concerned with the so-called moving-target problem: the item studied is likely to change even as the evaluation is in progress. The most dynamic technologies often evoke the greatest controversy and require the most careful evaluation, but research methods will have to be adapted to allow for continuing change. Furthermore, the "moving-target" problem goes beyond the technology being studied. For example, changes in methods for diagnosing a medical problem can affect the assessment of a therapeutic procedure. Earlier detection of cancer can influence the results of evaluation of alternative therapies.[10]

A variety of federal agencies are currently involved to a greater or lesser extent in the evaluation of various types of medical technology, but there is neither commonality nor coordination to their efforts. As previously mentioned, the Food and Drug Administration (FDA) conducts premarketing screening of new drugs and, to a more limited extent, medical equipment. The National Institutes of Health (NIH) fund and conduct clinical trials as part of their research agenda, and their relative resource commitment to such activities has been increasing in recent years. These studies are undertaken in the context of a much wider research mission of the Institutes and are necessarily limited in scope. The Veterans Administration (VA) and the military medical system also support clinical trials, but because of their specialized patient populations, neither can generate all the information needed for the larger and more diverse civilian health care system. Other federal agencies conducting relevant assessment activities include the National Center for Health Services Research; the Center for Disease Control; the Alcohol, Drug Abuse, and Mental Health Administration; and most recently the National Center for Health Care Technology.

Over the past few years, several expert panels have examined the need for a systematic approach to generating and disseminating evaluative information on medical technologies. These groups have identified at least three alternative approaches to the problem.

The first is the creation of a new government agency with powers ranging from the purely informative — based on research and analysis — to full-scale premarketing regulatory authority similar to the FDA model. This latter approach, while both plausible and comprehensive, has major drawbacks, the most obvious of which is the possibility that any regulatory-style review could constrain innovation and significantly slow the diffusion of valuable new technology throughout the health care system. There is already considerable concern about the "drug lag" problem in the United States, which has been attributed to the existing FDA clearance procedures. Given the current antiregulatory mood in the United States, there seems little likelihood that either Congress or the executive branch would favor extension of regulatory authority to all types of medical technology. And even if that sentiment should change in the future, there would be considerable opposition to the creation of a wholly new agency for this purpose. In practice, it has traditionally been more feasible to extend the functions of one or more existing institutions than to create a new one.

A second approach to the assessment of medical technology is currently being pursued by the National Institutes of Health, which in 1977 launched a process of "consensus development" — the bringing together of research scientists, practicing physicians, consumers, and others in an effort to reach general agreement on the efficacy and safety of specific technologies. Although the emphasis was to be on scientific considerations, ethical questions and cost implications were also seen as potential subjects for discussion. Approximately two dozen such consensus development conferences have been held since the program began in September 1977, covering topics ranging from dental implants to treatable brain damage in the elderly. Three of the most widely reported conferences focused on the use of mammography for breast cancer screening in women, the role of electronic fetal monitoring, and two different types of intestinal bypass surgical procedures.[11]

A third approach has been suggested in an Institute of Medicine study.[12] The study committee viewed the NIH consensus development program as a useful step, but one whose value is limited by the paucity of hard evidence available to the experts who seek to judge various technologies. Beyond some point, authority simply cannot substitute for evidence. Interestingly, participants in the NIH consensus development groups have reached essentially the same conclusion. These groups have repeatedly stressed the need for more well-grounded empirical evidence about the efficacy, risks, and costs of technological innovations. The fact that many of the NIH panels failed to reach agreement because they lacked adequate information sharply highlights the need for such research studies.[13]

The Institute of Medicine study recommended an approach that would link research to the diffusion of a new medical technology, essentially by requiring all those who use a new technology to collect uniform data as a condition of reimbursement by third-party payers. This course has the merit of permitting rapid diffusion of promising new interventions while simultaneously gathering the hard evidence necessary for making well-informed judgments about the usefulness of the new tool. There are, of course, numerous questions to be worked out before such a system could be implemented. For example, who should identify the technologies to be screened? Who should draft the research protocols? Who should fund the studies? Who should evaluate the data? If guidelines of appropriate use are to be prepared, who should do so? To whom should the information be provided systematically?

The Institute of Medicine group that studied the diffusion of equipment-embodied technology recommended the establishment of a national coordinating body to accomplish most of these aims.[13] Its purposes would be the following:

1. To identify technologies that need to be evaluated.
2. To fund planning and evaluation studies where existing funding programs are not adequate.
3. To disseminate available information about new and existing technologies after the data have been collected and analyzed.
4. To improve methods for evaluating medical technology by sponsoring or conducting appropriate research.
5. To coordinate evaluative programs of federal agencies and possibly foster an international exchange of information.

This coordinating body need not be governmental. Alternatives include a nonprofit organization such as a council on technology supported by a consortium of public and private third-party payers. Wherever these functions are placed, it is important to achieve a major enlargement of the evaluative effort and not merely shift existing programs from NIH and VA, for example, to a new agency.

An enlargement of this research effort does not necessarily imply a net increase in health care expenditures, however. At present, third-party payers frequently reimburse for new procedures before their effectiveness has been definitely established. If in the future they were to reimburse only for new procedures conducted on their beneficiaries as part of evaluative research approved by the national coordinating body, we might well see a significant savings in medical costs rather than continual increases. With or without substantial cost savings, such an approach has the potential for contributing substantially to continuing, long-term improvement of health care in the United States — and very likely in other countries as well.

Since the preparation of the Institute of Medicine report, a government agency has emerged that is intended to address many of these functions. This is the National Center for Health Care Technology. It is a part of the well-established and highly respected Public Health Service. It is administratively placed in a cluster with two closely related agencies, the National Center for Health Statistics and the National Center for Health Services Research. The three agencies taken together are dwarfed by such better-known sister agencies — also part of the Public Health Service — as the National Institutes of Health and the Food and Drug Administration.

The new National Center for Health Care Technology has started on a very small scale, certainly not commensurate with the magnitude of its long-term tasks, but perhaps sufficient to build a foundation. Its ultimate fate can be regarded as highly uncertain at this early stage. In 1980, the center announced its intention to solicit research grant applications in seventeen priority areas, selected on the basis of recommendations from its advisory bodies, which include nongovernmental as well as governmental individuals. The priority group is as follows:

maternal serium alpha-fetoprotein test for prenatal detection of fetal neural tube defects
coronary bypass surgery
dental x-rays
total knee replacements
ultrasound for cardiac diagnosis
cerebral bypass surgery for treatment of stroke
positron emission transaxial tomography (PETT)
heart transplants
cardiac nuclear imaging
renal dialysis and kidney transplantation in end-stage renal disease
electronic fetal monitoring
computed axial tomography (CT scanning), head and body
barium enema
endoscopy in upper gastrointestional bleeding
skull x-rays
continuous flow analysis
electroencephalography

At current funding levels, it will take many years to mount definitive research in these seventeen areas, let alone in others that are emerging. Therefore, it seems prudent to view this list primarily as an assessment of what is needed.

Such research will inevitably confront the problem raised several years ago in an Institute of Medicine study of the standard of evidence to be employed in decisions about health care technology.[14] In discussing the evidence for establishing efficacy of CT scanning, the report said:

> In making specific recommendations about efficacy, the committee has based its judgments on the published literature. That literature shows the remarkable promise of CT scanning, both in its applications to the head and more recently, as scan times have been reduced, to a number of indications in the body. However, this evidence is not based on carefully designed, large-scale clinical trials. Therefore, the committee can reach two different sets of conclusions about efficacy at the level of diagnostic impact. The first would be based on existing standards of clinical evidence evaluated by the expert judgment of leaders in the field. Many significant advances in diagnosis and treatment have been introduced into practice on the basis of this type of evidence, and the results over time, when evaluated have shown very positive value. The second type of evidence would require clinical trials meeting high standards of experimental design and statistical significance. The evidence for CT scanning, even in the head, does not yet meet this second standard . . .. The policy recommendations can be very different, depending on which standard would call for a finding of diagnostic efficacy for CT scanning in the head and for a number of indications in the body. The second standard would find the results still inconclusive. The logical policy conclusion based on the first standard would be to recommend reimbursement for those uses found efficacious. The conclusion based on the second standard would be that the procedures are still experimental and should be supported only in settings that are part of a clinical trial leading to more definitive evidence. Only when that more definitive evidence is available would reimbursement in all approved treatment settings be available . . .. The issue of the evidentiary base for clinical practice high-lighted in this report will, we believe, become very significant in establishing reimbursement and health planning policies in the coming years.

About two-and-a-half years after this report was published, the dilemma was highlighted for the general public in a *New York Times* editorial entitled "The Riddle of the Nobel Scanner":

The award of a Nobel Prize to the developers of the CAT scanner last week rightly recognized a revolutionary advance in medical technology. It should also revive concern over whether the United States is using such new machines wisely.

The scanner is considered the greatest advance in diagnostic radiology since the discovery of X-rays. At a half million dollars each, plus several hundred thousand a year for operation, it is also very expensive. More than 1,100 CAT scanners have been sold in this country; 900 have been sold in the rest of the world. Should their further deployment in America be limited? Or has the medical profession passed the line of due regard for our increasing medical bills? . . . According to the Congressional Office of Technology Assessment, the machines were evaluated more carefully than many medical devices, yet they are widely deployed without detailed proof of their effectiveness or safety . . . . Nobody can be sure of how many CAT scanners are needed or where to locate them. As patients, we want the best possible care and hang the cost. As taxpayers and insurance subscribers, we want cost-effective care. Perhaps a new Nobel Prize can be offered to those who can solve such costly riddles.[15]

The issues involved in the linkage of technology diffusion with systematic research in health care are interestingly illustrated by the current emergence of a plausible new technique for opening up partially clogged coronary arteries. Since arteriosclerotic heart disease is so common and constitutes such an enormous burden of illness in industrialized countries, any procedure that offers promise of alleviating the disease process and its consequences is likely to spread rapidly, even in the face of formidable costs and risks.

A clinical report published in 1979 suggested that nonoperative dilation of stenosis could be achieved by a balloon catheter technique — essentially the passage of a tube into the diseased artery, then inflation of the balloon so as to flatten an obstructing lesion on the vessel wall and so increase blood flow to the heart. The report stated:

In percutaneous transluminal coronary angioplasty, a catheter system is introduced through a systemic artery under local anesthesia to dilate a stenotic artery by controlled inflation of a distensible balloon.

Over the past 18 months, we have used this technic in 50 patients. The technic was successful in 32 patients. 29 patients showed improvement in cardiac function during follow-up examination. Because of acute deterioration in clinical status, emergency bypass was later necessary in five patients; three showed electrocardiographic evidence of infarcts.

Patients with single-vessel disease appear to be most suitable for the

> procedure, and a short history of pain indicates the presence of a soft (distensible) atheroma likely to respond to dilatation. We estimate that only about 10 to 15 percent of candidates for bypass surgery have lesions suitable for this procedure. A prospective randomized trial will be necessary to evaluate its usefulness in comparison with surgical and medical management.[16]

In an accompanying editorial, the Director of the National Heart, Lung and Blood Institute (NHLBI) — a component of the National Institutes of Health — put the clinical report into useful perspective:

> The report provides evidence that in carefully selected and prepared patients, and in the hands of an experienced team, balloon angioplasty can effectively dilate highly stenotic coronary vessels and provide immediate improvement in myocardial perfusion and myocardial performance, as measured both subjectively and objectively. Moreover, this improvement can persist for six months or longer. Thus, percutaneous transluminal coronary angioplasty can be seriously considered as a promising new technic.
>
> However, even though the technic seems promising, caution must be exercised and the technic put into perspective. Even the skilled angiographer should not undertake the procedure unless he has been specifically trained. The physician who attempts the procedure must have a surgical team ready to perform immediate coronary surgery, if necessary. The patient must be prepared for surgery. As agreed unanimously at a recent meeting held in Bethesda and as discussed below the technic must still be considered investigational since its long-term effects, risks, indications and contraindications are still not fully recognized.
>
> Since the procedure is still in an investigational stage, any physician contemplating the use of the technic should first obtain approval from his institutional review board for the research protocol . . .. For the present there is clearly a need for careful collection and analysis of clinical experience and for prompt dissemination of this information to minimize adverse effects while taking advantage of the value of the technic. The responsibility should be shared by investigators, institutions and their review boards, and by the manufacturers of the devices.[17]

In a situation of this kind — and there are many — it is important to stimulate research rapidly, to pool information (e.g., through a registry of all cases), and to provide rapid feedback of results to practitioners and interested parties. This will require cooperation of research-sponsoring agencies and financing bodies — for example, the Public Health Service and the Health Care Financing Administration. The linkage of diffusion with research involves clinical, methodological, logistical, and ethical problems of formidable complexity. But there is no reason to assume they are insurmountable. They are now being examined in detail by the Institute of Medicine (a nongovernmental body) and by governmental bodies. Considerable progress may be anticipated in the next decade.

The closer linkage of health care research — such as biomedical technology assessment — to the quality of care can be accomplished in large part through academic health centers and professional bodies. The means of reaching these goals require analysis in the near future in light of escalating health care expenditures.[18] In pluralistic societies, there are important roles for nongovernmental institutions in strengthening health care research and linking it to the health services.

University-based health centers, for example, can probably contribute considerably more than they have in the past. In this connection, the following questions need further examination:

1. How is it possible to organize the functions of academic medical settings to improve the environment for health care research? Can useful lessons be learned from the strengthening of basic biomedical research after 1945?
2. How can the medical specialities be effectively linked with other pertinent university activities — e.g., engineering statistics, social sciences? What are the conditions favorable to long-term interdisciplinary research on health care — reaching beyond the medical center to communities of everyday life where appropriate? What relations of academic health centers and professional societies will foster rapid dissemination of reliable information on the uses of health care technology? These questions embody a challenge of great importance for the medical centers of the future and indeed for the quality and credibility of health services.

SUMMARY

The past few decades have seen a rapid acceleration of diffusion of well-intentioned, plausible interventions in diagnosis, therapy, and prevention. Though partly derived from scientific work at the laboratory bench, they have usually not been rigorously evaluated scientifically prior to widespread use. These interventions are often beneficial, but sometimes they fall far short of their putative benefits, may have considerable associated risks, and usually add to the cost of health care.

So, a powerful stimulus is emerging for strengthening clinical research and extending it, where appropriate, to large-scale research on health care per se — including questions of efficacy, safety, usefulness, cost, organization, and financing. But such research has not had a high priority in the past and poses formidable clinical, methodological, logistical, ethical, and financing problems. The linkage of such research to the initial diffusion of new health care interventions is a particularly significant arena for health improvement in the future. The crucial integrative task is to foster innovation and provide adequate assessment as rapidly as possible when innovation is applied to health care.

NOTES

1. U.S. Congress, Office of Technology Assessment, *Assessing the Efficacy and Safety of Medical Technologies* (U.S. Government Printing Office, Washington, D.C., 1978).
2. U.S. Department of Health, Education, and Welfare, Public Health Service, *Medical Technology: The Culprit Behind Health Care Costs? Proceedings of the 1977 Sun Valley Forum on National Health*, edited by S. Altman and R. Blendon (U.S. Government Printing Office, Washington, D.C., 1979). Also see Thomas W. Maloney and David E. Rogers, "Medical Technology — A Different View of the Contentious Debate over Costs," *New England Journal of Medicine* 301:1413-19, December 27, 1979.
3. Institute of Medicine, National Academy of Sciences, A Policy Analysis by a Committee of the Institute of Medicine, *Computed Tomographic Scanning*, April 1977.
4. Judith L. Wagner, "Toward a Research Agenda on Medical Technology," in *National Center for Health Services Research: Research Proceedings Series*, Urban Institute Conference, West Palm Beach, Florida, December 10-12, 1978 (U.S. Department of Health, Education, and Welfare, Public Health Service, Hyattsville, Md., September 1979).
5. Institute of Medicine, National Academy of Sciences, A Report by the Committee on Technology and Health Care, Assembly of Engineering, National Research Council and Institute of Medicine, *Medical Technology and the Health Care System*, 1979.
6. U.S. Congress, *Assessing the Efficacy and Safety.*
7. Institute of Medicine, *Medical Technology and the Health Care System.*
8. U.S. Department of Health, Education, and Welfare, Public Health Service, National Center for Health Services Research, *Research Proceedings Series*, Urban Institute Conference, West Palm Beach, Florida, December 10-12, 1978 (Hyattsville, Md., September 1979).
9. Wagner, "Toward a Research Agenda."
10. Ibid.
11. U.S. Department of Health, Education and Welfare, Public Health Service,

Office of Health Research, Statistics, and Technology, *Health United States — 1979* (Hyattsville, Md., 1979).
12. Institute of Medicine, *Medical Technology and the Health Care System.*
13. U.S. Department of Health, Education, and Welfare, *Health United States — 1979.*
14. Institute of Medicine, *Computed Tomographic Scanning.*
15. "The Riddle of the Nobel Scanner," *The New York Times,* Monday, October 15, 1979.
16. Andreas R. Gruntzig, Ake Senning and Walter E. Siegenthaler, "Nonoperative Dilatation of Coronary-Artery Stenosis, Percutaneous Transluminal Coronary Angioplasty," *New England Journal of Medicine* 301, no. 2, July 12, 1979.
17. "Percutaneous Transluminal Coronary Angioplasty," *New England Journal of Medicine* 301, no. 2, July 12, 1979.
18. Louis B. Russell, *Technology in Hospitals: Medical Advances and Their Diffusion* (The Brookings Institution, Washington, D.C., 1979). Also see Barbara Stocking and Stuart L. Morrison, *The Image and the Reality: A Case-Study of the Impacts of Medical Technology,* published for the Nuffield Provincial Hospitals Trust (Oxford University Press, Oxford, England, 1978).

Chapter 5

Disease Prevention and Health Promotion

Sir George Godber, D.M.

The great strides in medical technology before and during World War II gave many people — not least doctors — the impression that positive medical interventions offer the best hope for improving general health. Only recently have the escalation of health care costs and the recognition of treatment limits begun to rekindle interest in disease prevention and health promotion as ways of sustaining the health of the public.

DISEASE PREVENTION

The works of McKeown and the widely studied Lalonde Report on the Health of Canadians have made many people aware that disease prevention rather than treatment has been responsible for the great increase in life expectancy at birth in industrialized countries. The record of disease prevention reveals that there have been three main fields of action — first, control of potential hazards in the environment; second, promotion of better health habits, including nutrition at vulnerable periods of life, especially pregnancy; and third, specific interventions using drugs and vaccines to prevent or control particular diseases.

The preventive movement began in the middle of the nineteenth century before the development of microbiology revealed the causes of many infections that were the main causes of premature death. But the empirical approach through the removal of gross environmental pollution with human wastes was just as effective as it would have been after the identification of the human pathogens.

The program of environmental protection, pioneered in the last century, gradually extended into the regulation of many factors affecting both the home and the workplace. Such regulation has been substantially absorbed into area planning on the one hand and industrial regulation on the other. The simpler factors in hygiene are among the assumed provisions in any developed society, though they are all too often defective in developing countries, in urban and rural areas alike. The single most important requirement of a safe water supply is not yet available to a large part of the world's population, although it is a major feature in WHO's program. In most industrialized countries the basic services require maintenance, but the health services mainly require monitoring. Atmospheric pollution is still an important concern in industrialized societies, even though crude pollution by smoke, like industrial pollution of inland water, is controlled by services in which general health staff may play little part.

New hazards have arisen as the result of the great increase in the use of synthetic chemicals and in their discharge into the atmosphere and inland waterways after use in agriculture or as industrial wastes. A highly sophisticated monitoring system and alertness for relevant illness in the health services are both necessary, but the first is the main means of control. Major accidents have occurred from time to time as a result of accidental emissions into effluents of high intensities of toxic volatile chemicals or dusts or of the long continued discharge of metallic residues — for example, mercury compounds in Minimata Bay in Japan eventually reaching the human food chain in fish.

Uncertainty still exists about the effect of lead intake at a level too low for classical poisoning. In the last decade the monitoring of such discharges has been intensified, and long-term evaluation is still needed. The effect of lead derivatives used in petrol to secure more complete combustion has been suspect but not certainly incriminated in harm to health, though its critics are vociferous. The use of lead additives may prevent the emission in vehicle exhausts of incompletely burnt hydrocarbons that might be even more damaging.

Cadmium, cobalt, tin, asbestos, and a large number of compound chemicals have been found in wastes, as have radioactive materials, and rightly controlled on general grounds. The use of ionizing radiations has been controlled in both medical and industrial use for similar reasons. Many of these problems require careful balancing of benefits and disadvantages. We need expert monitoring and a balanced judgment between benefits and dangers. Such judgments often have to be made under pressure from vociferous and only partly informed comment in the media.

Particular circumstances may produce exceptional risks to groups of workers or to the public. Close monitoring of workers using new chemicals in industry and agriculture requires an expertise few possess, and some adverse effects, especially carcinogenesis, may appear very late. The example of the effect of naphthylamine producing bladder cancer in rubber workers is well known. In exceptional circumstances the normal exposure of workers may be greatly exceeded, and such exposure may even occur in the public as a result of unrecognized contamination of products, accidents in transit, or major accidents at production centers. Such events are reported at intervals in the world press, despite strict conditions of inspection under statutory regulations at plants. Pressure groups, despite their real value in some contexts, might urge such restriction by governments as would prevent other public gains, but public acceptance is a prerequisite of, for example, the use of nuclear sources of power. The balance between an almost infinitesimal risk of a major disaster and short-term but general gains needs open assessment rather than blind acceptance of expert judgments that may be made from too narrow, however elevated, a base.

Improved safety of public water and food supplies, as well as a more nearly sufficient supply of both, may have been the largest factor in reducing illness and premature death in the first half of this century. The abundance of food may have gone too far in some through encouraging overweight, despite the desperate shortages in too many others. The food industry, in sophisticating its products, has often pandered to and even promoted an unsatisfactory balance of nutrients. Some affluent countries have increased the refined carbohydrates in their diets at the expense of recontaining cereal foods. The saturated fat and cholesterol content of some diets has been increased at the expense of vegetable fats, with a higher proportion of polyunsaturated fatty acids.

Unfortunately, there is no consensus among experts on the adjustments that are needed, save on the avoidance of excess. We need better guidance on nutrition and strictures on industry's promotion of the wrong kind of foods. Nevertheless, the greater part of the world's population is rightly concerned to obtain the sufficiency of food that it now lacks. Only Norway seems to have propounded a food and agriculture policy on lines intended to promote health.

Certain new factors in food supplies affect their safety. Synthetic chemicals are used at various stages in the food chain for the treatment of seed corn, as pesticides or herbicides in production and storage, as "improvers" in presentation for sale, as coloring, or as preservatives. National and international monitoring and supervision by experts is needed, backed by statutory authority for enforcement. Chemicals used as fertilizers may have remote effects such as nitrification of water supplies to a level that might endanger susceptible infants through public water supplies. Nitrites used in the preservation of meat may help in the formation of minute amounts of nitrosamines, which are carcinogenic at higher concentrations, but if used at too low a concentration may allow anaerobic organisms such as that causing botulism to grow in the meat. This last is an excellent example of the need for a careful balance of arguments for and against substances and processes.

The DeLaney clause in U.S. food and drug legislation is written in such uncompromising terms that it might have stopped the use of sweetening agents, leading to a far more damaging use of sugar, had not Congress intervened. On the other hand, failure to ensure strict control of the use of antibiotics in animal husbandry may have helped the emergence of resistant strains of human pathogens.

Knowledge that misuse of chemicals can have disastrous results has sometimes caused great alarm among the public. That partly explains the frequently successful resistance to one of the simplest, safest, and most certainly effective procedures in public health — the fluoridation of water supplies for the prevention of dental caries. New Zealand and the Republic of Ireland have laws requiring the fluoridation of reticulated water supplies; the United States has encouraged the practice and achieved about 50 percent success; Britain has achieved barely 10 percent success; and Sweden has even legislated against it.

All countries need systems for obtaining dispassionate advice from experts and adequate public information and consultation. The example of the U.S. Institute of Medicine within the National Academy of Sciences is especially interesting in this regard. Other countries have other systems, notably the Netherlands, France, Britain, and Sweden, but in principle, expertise and independence are essential requirements, with full public participation and involvement.

The development of personal health care as a preventive measure began with mothers and young children, usually in the form of screening examinations and advice. Three-quarters of a century of such work has produced a generation with better understanding of children's needs. The services now tend to concentrate on women with known or suspected abnormalities in pregnancy and childbirth, though with a strict routine supervision for all, and on children with known adverse factors at birth or in their families. Recognition of the importance of early and sustained antenatal care and the secondary requirement of occasional expert intervention during delivery have reduced maternal mortality by more than 90 percent in the last forty years. A maternal death is now a rare event in an industrialized country. But there are appreciable differences between such countries in neonatal mortality, which is closely linked to variations in the prematurity rate.

There is every reason to maintain pressure for improvement in care for the pregnant woman and neonate. Countries vary in their systems of maternity care. Most of those represented at Salzburg provided for more than 90 percent of deliveries in hospital, but in the Netherlands at least half the deliveries take place at home. Countries vary also in their use of midwives, some expecting obstetricians or family doctors to undertake most deliveries. The Netherlands has a unique service of highly trained midwives who work in patients' homes in a more independent role than those of Britain, where most deliveries are also supervised by midwives but in hospital. Discussion at Salzburg left the impression that most countries have movements in favor of reducing the institutional aura surrounding birth, but that this could be achieved by different handling of patients by institutional staff. The Netherlands' view of the advantages of home delivery was stressed, but there was no clear evidence about costs, which were thought to differ little between the two systems. The choice should be made on relative risks and maternal preference, but there is little chance of a properly controlled trial in present circumstances. The notable reduction in neonatal mortality in France during the 1970s appears to be the outcome of a campaign to improve antenatal and neonatal care, including making cash allowances conditional on attendance for antenatal care. It seemed that too little attention had been given to the opinions of women themselves, with full information and adjustment of management in accordance with their wishes.

Preventive services for children derive from programs of routine examination in infancy and through school life. Some of these involve a large use of medical time, as in the USSR, without proof of benefit. Careful pediatric assessment at birth should be standard, and subsequent developmental assessment should make it possible to secure treatment at the most advantageous time if abnormality is found. Some screening procedures are certainly advantageous when they bring children with disabilities such as hearing loss, cardiac abnormalities, hip dislocation, or squint promptly to treatment at the time of detection. The trend in recent years has been to identify those children needing special attention. Nurses and other health professionals may be able to provide a better screening service, supplementing the essential medical component, than could be provided by physicians alone. This is especially true of early problems of management in which child psychologists or psychiatrists may be able to help in a supporting role. The need to admit children to hospital has become less frequent, and the role of the hospital-based pediatrician can be exercised in support of primary care from a family doctor, though in North America and Sweden many children receive primary care from pediatricians, and in the USSR this is the rule.

In the USSR a system known as dispensarization has been used to supervise the health of adult groups, particularly those who have had hospital treatment or women after delivery. In North America the practice of annual physical checkups for apparently healthy adults has been widely followed — indeed, it is one of the great differences in family practice between the two countries and Britain. Some groups in Britain have elaborated such procedures by adding an array of laboratory and radiological checks, comparable to those used in multiphasic screening. This process has been used outside the National Health Service mainly for senior executives. Its value like that of other checkup systems can only be described as unproved, although a recent assessment for the U.S. Institute of Medicine of multiphasic health testing gave a guardedly favorable view.

Clinics for periodic review of older people have been established under various auspices. Since some pathology, which may be remediable, is commonly present, such clinics may have a use. A better method may be an annual check, at least by older patient reporting. Some family doctors do this and report subjectively favorable outcomes. At the least this method reduces the risk of social isolation of an old person and at best may bring him or her to treatment or rehabilitation at an early and remediable stage. If general practice is to provide continuity of care, this seems a valuable method. It is clearly most easily accepted within a resource ceiling in those services that do not depend on a fee per service system of payment. It also lends itself well to use by a primary health care team that includes nurses.

Population-screening programs of many kinds have had a vogue, more or less lasting, in recent years. The earliest and most important introductions involve prenatal recognition of conditions that may require action. An early example was serological testing for syphilis, which has largely prevented congenital syphilis as well as enabling the cure of the mother. Blood grouping, Rhesus typing, and haemoglobin estimation are part of the routine of antenatal care. Rhesus sensitization should be detected and can affect treatment, but use of anti-D globulin at the time of delivery can prevent sensitization from occurring. The more recent development of testing for fetal abnormalities by amniocentesis at sixteen weeks of pregnancy in high risk cases makes possible termination of an abnormal pregnancy in societies that accept such action. Termination is now undertaken in many countries for risks to the mother or fetus; this has certainly saved the lives of many who might never otherwise have resorted to illegal intervention. The ethical problems were discussed in other contexts at Salzburg.

Neonatal assessment and later developmental assessment are a progressive screening system in themselves. Their emphasis is not so much on point of time measurements, such as visual acuity, as on functioning and progress. Some screening is used in immunization programs, but mass screening of populations was first used in miniature radiography for pulmonary tuberculosis. Mass radiography is now used selectively in industrialized countries only for groups at special risk, but the reduction from whole population screening was often resisted as if it implied a deprivation from a particular good rather than the end of a need. Habit formation and illusions of persecution seem to develop as easily in the public as in the professions over rituals once established.

Screening for cancer of the uterine cervix was the next program on a comparable scale, though not, of course, for the whole population. Some countries, such as Britain, have tried to reach only a vulnerable age group at a moderate frequency, others have offered a more frequent service to all ages. The argument on policy is complex, but this is a good example of the need to keep technology within bounds. There is still dispute about the benefits, and there is a group subject to the highest incidence of the disease that is the least accessible to screening. The volunteers tend to be those who need the service least.

Screening for breast cancer by mammography with or without palpation and thermography has been subject to one major trial and developed in some form on a limited basis, but proof of widespread benefit as opposed to mere accuracy of identification is limited. The question is still open, and a recent appraisal for the National Academy of Sciences was moderately favorable. Screening for hypertension might become of greater importance, since the severe forms should be under treatment and would benefit. Public demand might surpass medical enthusiasm, as for some other forms of screening. Screening for diabetes seems justifiable only if targeted, but screening for raised intraocular tension is insufficiently specific or sensitive for the control of glaucoma. In special vocational situations, as in air pilots, intensive screening for coronary artery disease may be justified.

At Salzburg, we touched upon the ethical problems and seemed more inclined to favor selective screening within family practice with a certainty of followup than populationwide searches, which might alarm excessively and overload treatment services with patients falsely reported positive. This does not mean that all family practices were believed to function in this way. Certainly screening without the possibility of treatment, if required, was thought wrong.

By comparison with the present, the pioneers of public health in the last century were handling crude biological hazards upon which they could pronounce from their own knowledge. Environmental protection today still requires local trained executants, but a far more sophisticated scientific monitoring and advisory system is also required at national and international levels.

A somewhat similar but even more recondite provision is needed to control the safety of drugs. Most drugs and biological products now used in medicine afford benefits far greater than the drugs they succeeded, but they also impart new risks. Their very effectiveness reduces the margins within which they must be used in man. Therefore, every country wishes to use them, but must be sure of the safety and quality of those it uses. It is usual to have an expert national supervisory body to require testing and to set the limits it can impose or have imposed by a statutory licensing body. But safety of drugs requires a continuous process of quality control that must be subject to oversight during manufacture. Sampling of the product is insufficient by itself. Some adverse effects can only be detected as a result of continuous monitoring of reports by users over long periods of time and extensive use. A somewhat different problem of the overuse of drugs is often attributed to aggressive marketing by producers. Whatever the apportionment of responsibility, the Seminar was well aware that a high and probably excessive part of the resources available for health is spent on drugs. The abuse of dependence-producing drugs is a different but major problem in most industrialized societies.

Specific prophylactic procedures began with vaccination against smallpox, a procedure that has now made possible, under WHO auspices, the elimination of a highly communicable and commonly lethal disease. The vaccine was a living virus derived from an allied bovine infection. It produced a local lesion and a humoral immunity against the generalized human disease. Other vaccines have been developed during this century from modified toxins or the bodies of killed or attenuated organisms, both bacteria and viruses. Their use is not wholly devoid of risk, but the chance of an adverse effect from those in use routinely in childhood is minimal in comparison with the possible effect of a natural infection.

Most countries now use schedules of immunization during childhood that should protect the child against most of the former serious, specific infections of childhood. Whooping cough, tetanus, diphtheria, poliomyelitis, measles, and rubella in girls, and sometimes BCG against tuberculosis in susceptibles of either sex, make up the usual sequence. If all these vaccines were fully effective and fully used, the diseases would only occur if imported. No one achieves such a result for three reasons: first, one of the vaccines — whooping cough — is not 100 percent effective and occasionally causes some adverse effects that are usually transient; second, measles is seldom a severe illness in older children, and the vaccine itself may produce a very mild illness; third, some parents are still uncertain of the value of protection to their children. There are risks of serious effects with some of these vaccines to perhaps one child in a quarter of a million to a million vaccinated. What would have happened to such susceptible children in a natural infection might have been a great deal worse, but that cannot be proved. In many countries, therefore, there are still some children who could be saved from illness by a complete vaccination program and a few from death.

The failure to achieve completeness in a vaccination program is possibly due to ineffective exposition to parents who have been exposed to some grossly exaggerated presentation of the supposed risks by people who are undoubtedly genuine but misinformed. As an example, highly misleading presentation of the level of risk by both medical and lay personalities in Britain reduced the success of the whooping cough immunization by half. As the number of susceptible young children increased, two years later the incidence of the disease — almost entirely among the unimmunized — increased more than tenfold, and the number of deaths fivefold. More effective programs could still save much illness and a few lives.

Paradoxically, there are also vaccines against such diseases as typhoid, paratyphoid, cholera, and influenza that are much in demand, although they are known to be of doubtful efficacy unless carefully chosen. Safety from the three enteric infections is ensured by clean water and food rather than by vaccines. Safety from influenza cannot be guaranteed by any vaccine yet available. In the light of recent Swine flu experience in the United States, it must be doubted if any health administration would choose to launch the population it serves upon such a medical adventure as mass immunization against influenza with the vaccines we have now. The epidemic behavior of the disease is so variable and the virus strain variation so abrupt that prediction is extremely hazardous.

It was recognized at Salzburg that preventive measures have received too little emphasis in health programs. Funds should be found for them, but preventive programs should undergo no less critical evaluation than treatment, though by different measures. They have not always been subject to such scrutiny, particularly in screening for inapparent disease and in the use of some vaccines.

Evaluation should be applied to existing programs as to some long-established treatments. For example, some countries still require entrants to be vaccinated against smallpox, and some continued routine vaccination of infants years after others had judged that the success of the WHO eradication campaign justified abandoning it. The extent to which routine health checks are undertaken varies between countries. They, too, must be seen as of uncertain value and require validation. The extreme example of dispensarization practiced in the USSR seems to be based on assumption rather than proved value. There seemed no basis for assessing the proportion of a national health budget that should be assigned to prevention, especially having regard to the fact that much prevention is best undertaken through those engaged in other forms of health care or in activities not necessarily regarded as "health" at all.

HEALTH PROMOTION

Having considered so far specific actions intended to prevent specific ills, it is now necessary to consider, first, if there are factors in lifestyle or other circumstances that could promote better health, and second, how people could be persuaded to adopt them. There are certainly several factors in the common lifestyle in developed countries that are potentially harmful of which the most clearly identifiable are smoking and the abuse of alcohol. The incrimination of tobacco and alcohol is so clear and so well documented that they might have been included in the earlier review of toxic exposures. Research Paper 23 of the National Institute of Drug Abuse discusses, with a wealth of detail, smoking as a dependence process. But smoking and the use of alcohol have been so woven into the pattern of life in most European and American countries that we have to regard their use as still within the spread of normal behavior. That is changing for smoking, which is most clearly incriminated as a cause of illness and premature death because of its almost specific relationship with lung cancer and heart disease.

Without complicating the issue with too many figures, it is sufficient to say that the abolition of smoking would within a short time produce the largest reduction in morbidity and premature mortality that could result from any health-promoting activity open to us. Nearly thirty years of campaigning has arrested what was a steadily increasing trend. Now in Britain in the last six years the proportion of men smoking has fallen by nearly one-seventh, to 45 percent. In the United States, the proportion has fallen rather more, to 30 percent. A smaller but appreciable reduction has occurred among women. The most encouraging feature in Britain was that the largest fall occurred in males ages sixteen to nineteen. In both Britain and the United States, as in some other European countries, smokers are now a minority group among adults, both male and female.

Smoking deserves special attention, not only because it is the largest certainly avoidable hazard but also because it illustrates the difficulties of health promotion by traditional means. There is now an enormous literature about smoking and health, and there have been four world conferences and repeated resolutions by the World Health Assembly on the subject. Yet the holocaust continues, supported by a powerful and sustained international, commercial and sometimes governmental sales effort. Reason is clearly not enough. No doubt most smokers in Western Europe and North America known they run risks. At least half of the smokers want to stop and may have tried to do so.

Alcohol presents different problems, because, unlike tobacco smoking, its consumption is not a minority, but indeed a large majority, activity among adults. There is unequivocal evidence that any smoking is harmful, but that only excessive taking of alcohol is damaging. Thus, we have to try to persuade people to reduce their intake below some limiting amount we may choose for a day's consumption. However much I may personally wish alcohol was not used at all, I cannot postulate that as a requirement for optimum health. There is unequivocal justification for requiring restraint in the use of alcohol by drivers and even more by public service drivers. Perhaps the best hope would be to persuade people to adopt a limit such as three drinks a day, provided this did not become a standard intake for all. Somehow we have to escape from the swaggering enunciation of some for higher consumption as evidence of virility. There is no merit in being intoxicated or even in having been so. So far as alcohol and driving are concerned, governments should look to the realism of Sweden and cease restricting the giving of controlling tests by police as Britain does. The British record of road deaths compares well with that of other countries, but accidents of all kinds are still the cause of one-eighth of the lost years of working life among men in Britain, and driving after drinking contributes largely to that. Stern action could reduce road deaths by a third if it eliminated drink with driving.

No one can realistically suggest the prohibition of alcohol or tobacco in countries where they have by custom been allowed for so long. That would be a real infringement of personal liberty. But something must be done to curb promotion and to limit the freedom of the producers if governments are serious about health promotion. It is absurd to expect health agencies operating on insufficient budgets to engage in advertising confrontations with immensely wealthy industries that employ the most skilled propagandists in the business. The figures for a recent year in the United States show $6 million spent on the health message against smoking with $120 million spent on subsidies of various kinds to industry and $600 million spent by industry on tobacco promotion. We have no idea of the extent to which a good health promotional program could reduce smoking or the abuse of alcohol because those pushing the wrong message so consistently drown the right. Only governments can do what is required — and that means governments as a whole, not just their health ministries. Some governments have faced their responsibilities in this regard, mainly those in Scandinavia and, over smoking, the Republic of Ireland. But others still engage in the tobacco business themselves. The Seminar seemed generally of the opinion that the time for shilly shally was over; governments should act.

The problem of nutrition and overweight was discussed earlier. It links with the need for exercise and with the lack of opportunity for many city dwellers to take it. Some countries have natural resources for outdoor recreation more readily available than others. Some have a tradition of fostering such activity in organized breaks in working time. Most need to provide greater encouragement and facilities that need not be elaborate, but must be inviting and safe. Competitive athletics attract resources where simpler provision for the average person does not. Indeed, provision is far more likely to be of a kind to encourage convivial eating and drinking and even smoking in exactly the pattern the middle-aged overweight man does not need. The simple exercise of jogging has attracted enormous numbers in some countries, and bodies like the British Sports Council in cooperation with the Health Education Council have tried to encourage it. In the USSR there is extensive use of holiday facilities linked with work.

There are many fragments of health education that fit into both the health-caring and educational services. Health educators, therefore, need to see themselves as orchestrating a program in which others may most commonly present the message. Children should receive more information about health in the course of general education, which means that teachers must be provided with material to be used in their own ways. More could be done to recruit support through informed nonprofessionals in the community, such as the block health workers in the USSR. The Open University in Britain has established courses for nonprofessionals with this object, but their reach is naturally to thousands rather than to millions.

At Salzburg, we did not pursue this subject in detail, but were concerned with some general principles that seemed to have been neglected in national programs. It is useless to preach to the public about choosing more favorable lifestyles and then leave them to a real life situation in which it is far easier to opt for those that are unfavorable. Advertising and other forms of sales promotion are far more likely to urge smoking, drinking, riding, and consumption of sugar and fat than exercise, uncompetitive driving, the consumption of whole grain cereal foods, and avoidance of smoking or excess alcohol. The advertisers who drown the right message by sheer volume are the first to protest against the invasion of personal freedom if their own activities are restricted. There are always literary hacks willing to provide articles deriding health promotional activities, and they never lack prominent positions in the media.

If governments seriously want their people to be more healthy, they must stop or limit those who want to sell them the wrong products, including themselves. If leaders of the health professions really want to reduce the load of curative work, they should apply themselves to active prevention. The Royal College of Physicians of London published the first major report on smoking and health in 1962 and followed it with two others. At the middle of 1979, the college still did not have No Smoking notices in its beautiful modern building. It has some polite requests now, but no prohibitions.

The general public is not about to be regulated into better health. It needs sensible leadership with balanced presentation of a good health message and a lot more coherence among the messages. Canada, the United States, Norway, Sweden, and Finland have been more active than some others, but there are few who do not make some attempt now. Too many countries seem to look to preventive medicine for short-term economies. The consensus at Salzburg was for the long-term aim. Action on that must come from governments, and health departments alone cannot make it effective. For that reason the WHO Expert Committee on Smoking Control and the 4th World Conference on Smoking and Health addressed their urgent representations to governments and not just to health ministers. The fellows at the Seminar would have applied that to other fields as well. Yet none of this emphasis on governments will be effective unless the health professionals recognize their own individual duties to contribute to the same end. The primary health care team is probably the most important of all.

CONCLUSION

The great increase in life expectancy at birth of 40 percent or so that occurred in most developed countries in the first half of this century has been followed by thirty years or so in which the improvement has been small, perhaps 5 percent. The figures lie in most industrialized countries between sixty-eight and seventy-two years at birth for males and seventy-three to seventy-seven years for females. The comparable figure for both sexes in 1900 was of the order of fifty years. But most of the gain is the result of reduced mortality in infancy and childhood. At age sixty-five the increase in life expectancy has been very small indeed, either for men or for women. The striking change in demography is that the proportion of babies who will survive to age seventy has more than doubled.

Without conceding that reduced mortality and increased longevity are more important advances than improved quality of life, it is important to consider what are the conditions from which mortality might be reduced. Banham devised an interesting presentation to the British Royal Commission on the National Health Service for this purpose with the title "Identifying Major Health Opportunities in Canada, the United States, Sweden and the United Kingdom." In a somewhat similar exercise in 1974, Hetzel compared Australia and England and Wales, using Sweden as the baseline. Banham constructed a mythical "Healthland," which had the most favorable mortality experience from among the four countries from grouped causes of death at ages one to five and then in decennia to sixty-five to seventy-four, separately for the sexes. That leaves Healthland with certainly avoidable mortality — for instance, it has the lung cancer mortality of Sweden, which all know is 90 percent avoidable — but with a level of achievement one of the four countries has made. Classification is assumed to be the same in each country between the groups. Each of the four countries is then compared with Healthland, and a rate of excess mortality is calculated for each age group and each disease group. It is refreshing that Britain actually has the smallest excess at ages fifteen to thirty-four, but thereafter the record is progressively worse. At ages sixty-five to seventy-four the excess mortality per 100,000 is 1680 for men and 775 for women compared with 1260 for men and 536 for women in the United States, 713 and 265 in Canada, and 345 and 242 in Sweden. Heart disease, cerebrovascular disease, lung cancer, and cirrhosis of the liver account for three-fifths of the excess for American men and women at all ages from thirty-five to seventy-four. For Britain the excess is mainly due to heart and cerebrovascular disease, chronic obstructive respiratory disease, and lung cancer, together accounting for three-quarters of the excess.

Since so large a part of this excess mortality is due to the known avoidable factors of smoking and abuse of alcohol, prevention is clearly possible — or would have been possible during earlier life. This method identifies for each of the four countries areas in which improvement should be possible in every age group — motor accidents in the United States and Canada, suicide and cirrhosis in Sweden, and mortality at the beginning of life in all but Sweden. It does not bring out how much even the best of the four might improve in each category, but it asks of the others no more than one has done.

Such methods also demonstrate that prevention now, apart from accidents and suicide, will mainly be of conditions with a long lead time. This is the crucial point in modern preventive medicine; the results will favor present younger generations in their future lives. Specific technical, medical intervention is rarely effective in prophylaxis of such diseases, but different patterns of behavior through early and middle life should enable those who adhere to them to live not merely longer, but healthier lives. In Chapter 6, on care of the elderly, I mention the observed higher standards of health and much increased life expectancy in those who do follow relatively simple good health practices in nutrition, avoidance of smoking, and modest or no use of alcohol as compared with those who do not.

It is, of course, impossible to know how far postponement of the onset of chronic degenerative or malignant disease is an economy for the health services of a nation. The avoidance of early death may lead to greater direct health care costs through a longer life. On the other hand, Luce and Schweitzer calculated that the costs of all kinds related to smoking and the abuse of alcohol would total about half as much as is spent in the United States in a year on health care. But a monetary basis is hardly appropriate to an assessment that must be made in human terms.

It is not to be expected that a successful program of prevention and health promotion would end with a large increase in life expectancy within the foreseeable future, if at all. If Britain and the United States were to abandon smoking wholly and now, it would still take some ten to fifteen years to produce the gain of some two years for men and half a year for women that would bring them to the position already enjoyed by Sweden. Our posterity does not seem likely to face prolongation of life by 10 percent by the end of the century or within a foreseeable interval after that. Whether or not there is an inextendable natural span that we are already approaching is uncertain, but the substantial difference between the highest and lowest socioeconomic groups in Britain suggests that considerable gain is still possible in reduced mortality and presumably in the quality of life, if we will simply commit ourselves to the implementation of more healthful policies and habits.

Chapter 6

Enabling the Elderly to Continue Functionally Independent

Sir George Godber, D.M.

THE SIZE OF THE PROBLEM

The world's population has grown rapidly during this century, especially in the last thirty years, for four main reasons — the increase in food supplies; the improvement in environmental hygiene leading to a reduction of diseases spread by water and food; the control of various other infectious endemic and epidemic diseases in childhood; and the control of tuberculosis.

These four factors have operated at different times in different countries. Though a large part of the world's population still lives in countries where they have been insufficient if not largely inoperative, these factors have been sufficiently effective in industrialized countries for long enough to have produced broadly comparable situations.

Already in Britain and Sweden more than one-seventh of the population is aged over sixty-five and in the United States the portion is about one-ninth. In Britain there were estimated to be some eight million people aged sixty-five and over in 1979, making up 14.5 percent of the population. The number will increase slowly to some 8.25 million within ten years and remain at that level until it falls back to the present level by the end of the century, if present mortality levels continue.

About 23 percent of boys and 26 percent of girls born in 1841 survived to 1911 — seventy years. Of babies born in 1975, even without further reductions of mortality in childhood and adult life, 58 percent of boys and 75 percent of girls should survive to the year 2045. In the United States, according to the Bureau of the Census, 12.2 percent of the population will be over sixty-five by the year 2000 and 18.3 percent by 2030.

The number of very old people will increase, while the numbers at ages sixty-five to seventy-four, already at a peak, will decline. In the next ten years the number aged seventy-five to eighty-four will increase by a third of a million, or about one-eighth, while the number aged eighty-five and over increases by a quarter and in the ensuing ten years by another fifth. Other industrialized countries differ slightly from this pattern because of past differences in birth rates, but all will have more elderly and, especially, more very old people.

Life expectancy has increased more for women than for men. There is now a gap of from four to seven years. Inevitably, then, the very old now include a large proportion of women who lack the mutual support between spouses that helps old people to live independently. Almost two-thirds of British men aged seventy-five to eighty-four live with their wives, but less than a quarter of women of that age group live with their husbands.

SOME COMMON AFFLICTIONS OF AGING

The figures presented above are often used loosely, as if the young and productive were about to be engulfed by decrepit elderly whose care they must assume. It is true that the old, like the very young, make heavier calls on the health and social services than do those in the normal years of working life. Much of this is due to the increased incidence of chronic degenerative and malignant disease at later ages.

There is some information about one of the most troublesome problems in care of the elderly, senile dementia. Dementia quickly destroys the individual's capacity to live independently and, if it continues, will exceed the capacity of a surviving spouse and even more of other family members to manage in a household. The future management of the very old will depend on the proportion of them in which mental precedes physical deterioration. The elderly experience other mental illness just as do younger people, and it can be managed in the same way. Dementia, however, is the special problem of the age group, and if it can be limited or its onset and development postponed, the individual and his or her family will benefit enormously, and the load on the community will be less.

A sample survey in northeastern England nearly twenty years ago suggested that 2.5 to 3 percent of those aged sixty-five to seventy-four might show "chronic brain syndromes" — not necessarily fully incapacitated — but that proportion doubled in the next five year age group and reached 20 percent in those aged eighty or over. We badly need to know if those proportions are representative and if they are still true. It is known that the age-specific rate for admission to psychiatric hospital care in Britain has fallen appreciably for people over seventy in the interval, though whether this is due to a reduced need or a greater neglect is not known. Physical deterioration and death must ultimately occur to everyone who escapes acute fatal disease, but postponement of mental deterioration until nearer that event would make care of even more of the elderly in the community far more practicable.

It is common knowledge, and documented in detail, that physical disabilities grow more numerous and more severe as age advances. There are wide individual differences, but unless some lethal episode such as myocardial infarction or malignant disease intervenes, all must eventually suffer more or less abrupt deterioration. The onset and progress of that deterioration may be delayed by many factors in the chosen lifestyle, social circumstances, and professional treatment or support. The determining factors long antecede the deterioration, and heredity may also be a major factor.

Various cross-section studies have shown that the proportion of old people suffering serious restriction of their social functioning increases rapidly with age. A survey in Britain found that almost three-quarters of the very severely handicapped needing special care were aged over seventy-five. Of the severely handicapped needing considerable support and the appreciably handicapped needing some support, almost two-thirds were in this age group. Taking these three groups as the disabled population, about two-sevenths of those over seventy-five were so classified. Admittedly only one-twentieth were in the very severe group, but that still leaves people over seventy-five needing far more health and social supports than any other age group. The picture, so far as it is known in other countries, is, unsurprisingly, much the same.

APPROPRIATE AND INAPPROPRIATE INTERVENTIONS

Some comment suggests that better health and social care has been used simply to prolong the lives of the aged through an ever-lengthening period of decrepitude and dependency. It appears to be assumed too often that during such an extended period of life, deterioration will occur at the same chronological age as thirty years ago. But it is not inevitable that deterioration of capacity for independence during a longer life will now start as early as in former times. Though the individual in his and more often her seventies will almost certainly require more services before reaching a preterminal phase of dependence than they required in their sixties, the major burden of irreversible dependence now falls later on the family and society.

It was generally agreed at Salzburg that the ideal situation for elderly people is continued independent living in their own homes, with at least their own familiar personal effects around them. This view commended itself to the fellows not only because a hospital bed is probably the most expensive place to maintain anyone, but because self-reliance is the best emotional and, therefore, somatic condition.

Of course, the most effective way to prolong capacity and independence is the maintenance of a healthy lifestyle in earlier years. The Alameda County studies by the University of California have shown that life expectancy in early middle age correlates closely with the way in which some simple "good health practices" have been followed. The seven good health practices studied were physical activity, regular meals, taking breakfast, using alcohol in moderation or not at all, avoiding smoking, ensuring sufficient sleep and preserving a reasonable height to weight ratio. Men forty-five years old who followed six or seven of these practices had a life expectancy of thirty-three years, compared with twenty-two years for those following three or less. Even more significant, if less precisely quantified, was the observation that at all ages, the "better" group had a physical status equal to that of men twenty to thirty years younger in the "worse" group. The difference for women, whose life expectancy is seven years greater than that of men, was less but in the same direction. Ten years later it was found that the lifestyle of the individuals, despite the publicity given to the findings, was hardly modified at all in either group.

Nevertheless, deterioration cannot forever be postponed. Its onset can, however, be staved off by more timely and appropriate interventions than are now in common use. The needs are of two kinds — procedures to arrest, cure, or alleviate disease by specialist treatments such as surgery for cataract, hypertrophy of the prostate, perineal repair, or hip joint replacement; and long-term relief ranging from domestic and nursing support in the home to continued medication or eventual accommodation in a welfare home or hospital for long stay care.

It is a grave error to think of the health and welfare needs of the elderly as being mainly for long-term care in hospitals or nursing homes for the physically or mentally ill. British statistics show that a quarter of all nonmaternity hospital admissions for physical illness are of patients aged over sixty-five and that just under half of these are ages seventy-five or over. But only one out of eleven of the sixty-five to seventy-four year old group and only two out of seven of the over-seventy-five group are admitted to geriatric departments for medium- or long-term care. In some other departments the average stay of these older patients may be longer — half as long again as the age group forty-five to sixty-four for general surgery — but in the main they need services of the same general nature as do younger people. Treatment for cataract, fractured femoral neck, malignant disease, or hip joint replacement may be mainly a requirement of the elderly, but the skills and technology required by the hospital staff are of the same general kind as are used for younger patients. It follows that the active medical interventions most commonly required by old people from hospital-based specialists involve only short hospital stays. Similarly, old people living at home suffer from the same short-term illnesses as others and require the same kind of help. Timely provision of appropriate help can often restore functional independence for many years.

There are many ways in which incapacity can be deferred, from the use of individual wealth to hire the maximum of support to the provision of home caring services from public funds. Family and neighborly supports are nontechnical and are overall the most important component in care. They are less likely to be available in a highly mobile than in a relatively stable society. Confidence will be strengthened if it is known that relief, temporary or permanent, will be available if breakdown occurs. Such supports include provision of homemaking help, both light and heavy; social visitation for isolates; nursing assistance in the home, with medical attendance as needed; other technical help such as physiotherapy, podiatry, provision of aids for hearing or vision; assistance with shopping and guidance on application for any entitlement; special provision for heating in winter; meals delivered to the home or available at social centers used for other social supporting activities; help with radio or travel; telephones or the means to pay for them; special housing and, if needed, oversight and assistance in it.

To maintain their independence, all people, not just the elderly, need access to primary care. Some countries, such as the Netherlands, Denmark, Britain, and New Zealand, have made general medical practice the gateway to their health care systems. Some, like the United States, Canada, and Sweden, accept that patients may seek primary care from specialists, mainly in internal medicine, pediatrics, and gynecology. All industrialized countries have some system that, for old people at least, finances consultation with primary physicians either from taxation (Britain, Poland, Sweden), insurance (Israel, most of the EEC countries, Canada, and Australia), or a special insurance arrangement made by government (United States). Technical medical care is, therefore, available, but there are considerable variations in the extent to which it is associated with other technical health inputs, such as nursing, and even more with the social supports.

Of course, for many people institutionalization cannot be avoided altogether. The disabilities of old people that make the heaviest calls on health and social services are those requiring long-term support, whether at home or in an institution. Of nearly 22 million days of care for the people over seventy-five in nonpsychiatric British hospitals, some two-thirds are in geriatric units or general-practitioner-supervised beds. Even at the age of sixty-five to seventy-four, one-third of the days of care are in geriatric units. These figures reemphasize the point that the elderly, and even more the very old, include a minority requiring care that is costly, because it is protracted, rather than requiring high technology support. The same point emerges in the United States, where some 1.1 million nursing home beds are in constant use. In Britain there are also twice as many places in welfare hostels as in geriatric units, and about two-fifths of the beds in psychiatric hospitals are used for patients over sixty-five — although not all for long stay care.

There are substantial differences in the way hospital care for the elderly is provided in different countries. Short-term care in which the needs of the elderly differ little from those of their juniors is the commonest requirement, and all countries handle this in much the same way. Some of the procedures are seldom required by the young — for instance, fixing a fractured femoral neck — but the essential nature of the surgical expertise and organization is not different. Nevertheless, rehabilitation of such older patients may require a slower tempo and greater persistence, and there are often social problems of home maintenance in which support is required. In some very old patients, the presentation of common acute conditions may be atypical, and there is often multiple pathology, not all of which requires the active intervention to which hospital activity is geared. A common complication of acute physical illness in the elderly is mental confusion, which will disappear with physical recovery but may complicate management in the hospital. Medical care of elderly patients requires continuity before, during, and after hospital stay.

Sweden has chosen to provide more of both hospital and hostel accommodation, currently enough to accommodate 14 percent of their population over age sixty-five. Denmark provides for some 8 percent, but has an interesting variant in care of the long stay chronically ill. Patients who have stayed three months in hospital and are not expected to recover sufficiently to go home are moved to nursing homes in which they live in rooms where they may have their own furniture. Essentially they are provided with homes for the rest of their lives to which any needed nursing, medical, or remedial resources are made available. The Danish elderly have a statutory right to such facilities. The homes are now all public and organized by the Social Welfare Authority. In the United States Medicare pays for nursing home care that involves much the same level of skill as those nursing homes of Australia that do not purport to offer technical services. There are large differences between countries in the scale of their provision and the degree of frailty of the residents, mainly dependent on the intensity of their effort to rehabilitate and return old people to their own homes and maintain them there.

THE ORGANIZATION OF SUPPORT SERVICES

While personal service and assisted or provided accommodation are obviously of great importance as the dependence of the most disabled minority increases, maintenance of income is the most important consideration for the elderly as a group. All developed countries have some system of social security payment to the elderly, as of right without demonstration of need, but the level of these cash supports varies widely. Some countries such as Denmark, West Germany, and the Netherlands have systems that ensure a generous competence for the elderly without proof of need. Others, like Britain, rely upon supplementary benefits to make good proven deficits. Given income maintenance at an adequate level, old people are much better able to make their own arrangements for support than in a society that allows too narrow a margin. If proof of need is required, there may be reluctance to provide it. The point recurred repeatedly at Salzburg that the ability to cope with today's situation must decline with age, just as the need for supports, including home management, increases. It was generally appreciated that a stereotype would not and should not be found, since each country must provide within its own customary social organization, but methods found successful in one country might point to possible modifications in another. The set of assumptions within which any country has designed its services should be constantly questioned and, where appropriate, modified.

Where services are required, nontechnical social supports are in many ways more necessary than medically oriented ones. Obviously, the family comes increasingly into the picture. Ideally the unit is the married couple, but the greater longevity of women, as previously indicated, and their earlier age of marriage means that the unit will more often be a lone woman than a lone man. In some societies it is still the custom for old people to live with their children. There are many reasons why this is less possible now. The old are older than at the beginning of the century, they have fewer descendants, and populations have become more mobile so that descendants live farther away. Despite the often repeated assertion that families are no longer willing to care for their elderly relatives, in Britain a higher proportion of people over sixty-five now lives outside institutions than at any earlier time in this century. Beyond family, the fit elderly, at an age when they might have been far more dependent in times past, constitute a resource for supporting the very old that has been used too seldom.

The fellows at Salzburg quoted different national patterns of ensuring social welfare supports. Most services seem to depend on user demand, which can vary for many reasons. There seemed a need in most countries to organize more deliberate intervention at an earlier stage, in whatever form may be found acceptable. Where there is a right not subject to a means test — as there usually is for social security payments — a service has no stigma attached to its acceptance and may be more readily used. Early intervention could be an important form of prophylaxis and in some countries extends to such paramedical inputs as physiotherapy, podiatry, and audiology. The basic essentials of adequate living space and supplementation of nutrition by meals either taken to the home or made available at special day centers or clubs are ensured to some by voluntary agencies or through local government. Grouped special housing is a feature in the Netherlands and West Germany. Accessibility to the ordinary amenities, shops, and libraries and visits from relatives are crucial but have sometimes been ignored as a result of very large aggregations of places in institutions chosen for administrative convenience.

Fellows at the Seminar presented information from their own countries on the best use of resources. The array of health and social supports — family care, community activities such as clubs and meal services, primary health care and social support through assisted special housing and hostels to day hospitals, outpatient hospital facilities, and acute or long stay inpatient care — is combined differently in different countries. Some of these differences are rooted in different social customs affecting the family, but there are also differences in professional community support systems, especially in primary health care.

Solutions to these problems vary — the simplest being the pragmatic British method of a separate specialty of geriatrics that does not limit the appropriate participation of the other specialties but does provide for the general care of the elderly. The method is specifically adjusted to the district organization of the British National Health Service and is not necessarily realizable elsewhere.

The speciality of geriatrics emerged forty years ago when a few internists working in large public hospitals began to concern themselves with the possibility of recovery for some of the large groups of elderly, chronically ill patients whose care had previously been largely custodial. These patients needed the application of no special technology other than that of internal medicine, but rather insight, persistence, and appreciation of their own and their families' needs. In some countries, such as Sweden, internists in the county hospitals already provided such care to some extent, but their solutions tended to keep many patients in the hospital who in Britain might have gone home. Thirty years ago it was still believed in Britain that internists or general physicians would take on the care of long stay patients. Indeed, the Royal College of Physicians produced a report only three years ago maintaining that this is their function. But they have seldom performed that task as effectively as the now large group of geriatricians does.

The special expertise required is social, and many internists not only lack it but are unaware that they need it to produce the best results for their patients. The geriatrician can assess the needs of old people with chronic illness or acute exacerbations for hospital care, manage their treatment and rehabilitation in hospital, and return most of them to their own homes to be supervised by the primary care team and to receive social welfare support if needed. Of course some patients die, and a smaller number are too disabled to be discharged and so remain in long stay wards. But the specialty is only effective if it fulfills an active role and handles most of its patients by active short-term care.

Naturally this specialty must work in conjunction with a home care medical and social welfare team, which has the responsibility for most of the frail elderly most of the time. It is a relief and technical support system using outpatient, day hospital, and inpatient facilities and providing a consultative service to the primary care team. It will be obvious that specially experienced nursing and good social service and rehabilitation staffs are essential to serve the same population. A team of professionals providing primary care must have mutual respect between its members and an awareness of the specific professional contribution that each can make. That is the objective of the British system, but there are often gaps and shortcomings in an arrangement that leaves each practitioner as an independent contractor.

A group at Salzburg discussed in some depth the way in which interprofessional relationships could be improved and systems of training made mutually more compatible, preferably with some common content. This has particular relevance to the care of the elderly, in which social as well as health professional supports can have a major effect on health maintenance. The group of health professionals comprises much more than nurses and physicians, but many of them work mainly in hospitals, whereas care of the elderly occurs mainly in the community.

The remedial professions are particularly important to the fullness of recovery from disabling illness. Early rehabilitation is even more important in the old than the young, whose natural resilience is greater. Pharmacists are an important and insufficiently used resource in the management of treatment of the elderly with drugs. The elderly are often asked to manage five or more different medications which, even if justified, they may confuse and misuse. There are many examples of primary care teams including a pharmacist, but few in which his or her professional skills are fully used in a consultative role with the physician or even as a readily available guide for the patient. The report of the recent Royal Commission in Britain has commented on this.

The group that discussed the elderly considered the financing of supports that could help surmount their problems. The prime requirement of sufficient income has been mentioned and the shortfall that in Britain requires supplementary payments by the Benefits Commission to one in four old people. Other supports are also best provided as of right without charge. Reliance on voluntary agencies for such services always carries the risk of gaps in different but related provision, and there are advantages in having a statutory local agency with an overall responsibility to ensure that a complete range of services is available. Even though such an agency may fail in detail, it is answerable for such failure and can be required to rectify it. That it does so in Britain, where there are parallel health and welfare authorities, is acknowledged in a recent report by Chapman on unmet needs in a part of London. Denmark has recently changed to a system that emphasizes the social needs even of long stay patients and makes one authority responsible for the complete range of long-term supports at home and in institutions.

The British Poor Law, dating back to the sixteenth century, was the historic pattern of public relief for the aged and destitute. This grew in the nineteenth century into a system of large institutions with negligible amenities. Their policies were, deliberately, minatory and their management niggardly, so that they were feared and avoided to the last by the aged poor. Since World War II these places have been largely replaced for welfare accommodation, but far too many of the buildings are still in use for the sick, with some, but insufficient, improvements. Smaller and more homelike hostels or group homes comparable with those that have been developed in Scandinavia and other Western countries have been provided. Private or voluntary homes provide some of the accommodation in Britain, but less than a sixth are in establishments run for profit.

Other countries make varying use of the voluntary or for profit homes. The Netherlands has a long tradition of using voluntary agencies in this field. Denmark used some independent homes, but now all that are used by public bodies are being taken over. The United States and Australia have relied heavily on so-called nursing homes. Finland makes state provision. The major policy difference between countries is the extent of the emphasis on returning old people to their own homes after a hospital admission. The intensity of development of support services in the community reflects this policy, which may be determined by human or economic considerations or a balance of the two.

SUMMARY

This discussion of needs and the ways in which they can be met is full of uncertainties. The needs have not been precisely ascertained, and they cannot be equated with demand, if only because the elderly may be least able to enunciate their demands. The individual presents a continuously evolving process rather than a single pathological state. The possible supports extend across a wide spectrum, and the means of deploying them vary with national custom and organization. Different cultures induce different attitudes in both the potentially supported and the potential supporters. The analysis can only be functional, matching services to the needs that can be defined; it is unlikely that there can ever be enough services if we succeed in identifying all the needs.

The formidable array of supports will only be provided if there is a sensitive system able to respond or even to act tactfully without direct request. Paul Chapman's study in the Pimlico area of London shows both how wide a coverage there can be and how it can fail through misinformation, inadvertance, or lack of funds. The best system searches out the most vulnerable isolates and identifies their needs. Either a primary health care team or a district social work service or the two together provide the best antennae and much of the support.

Whatever the local system of organization and the part played in it by volunteer agencies, it is essential that the elderly should play a part in determining what is to be done for them. Too little attention is given to the articulate handicapped and their views. Front line workers may hear, but the drift toward professionalization limits their freedom to help the elderly help themselves.

Chapter 7

Toward Regionalization in Health Services

Robert Maxwell

In recent years sweeping structural changes have been made in many health systems. As Petronius commented in the first century A.D., organizational change can unfortunately be a method of creating the illusion of progress without the substance.[1] Those who have lived through the trauma of major organizational upheaval may well share his cynicism, but the reasons are not always bad, and in the long run some of the changes will prove justified.

ASSESSING ORGANIZATIONS

The only real test of organizations is how well they work. In themselves they can achieve nothing. They are merely spaces better or worse designed for people to think and act. But that "merely" is not to be underestimated. For while a good structure is unnoticed, a bad one hampers action and narrows thought.

As described in Chapter 1 of this book, all health systems have evolved from a number of discrete, disjointed initiatives into a complicated web of sophisticated and expensive services. Today care often depends, far more than in the past, on how well several of these services work together. Moreover, the costs of duplication and of failure to cooperate are much greater than they were, and hard choices need to be made about how best to use limited resources. In these circumstances it is proper at least to question if the organizations that we have inherited are still appropriate.

Our answer to this question should, I suggest, be based on four criteria. The first is suitability for the particular purpose in hand, for "organization is a function of the work to be done."[2] Thus, we can assess a health system in terms of whether it promotes or hinders preventive activities and self-help, access to and continuity of care, and a sensible deployment and use of resources. Second is conformity with people's sense of what is appropriate and workable and with the talents available. An organization that works well in one culture will not work in another unless "it is in conformity with the deep-rooted sentiments of the men who have to make it work and thus productive of the requisite spirit and morale."[3] Third is simplicity and comprehensibility: other things being equal, the simpler the organization the better. People must be able to grasp and remember how it is supposed to work. Finally, and bottom of the list, is cost.

Judged against these criteria most health systems give no grounds for complacency. In countries where entrepreneurial activity is strong, as in West Germany and the United States, the disorganization of the system encourages duplication, institutional aggrandizement, and extravagance. Where systems are more tightly organized, as in Sweden, Britain, and Eastern Europe, there are dangers of bureaucratic sluggishness and overcentralization, staff disaffection, and falling standards.

SOME NATIONAL DEVELOPMENTS

From each of these two types of system, and from those in between, has emerged the theme of regionalization as a basis for reform. Indeed it is striking how widespread this theme is, arising apparently in many places simultaneously and independently. The roots of its appeal — and even its precise meaning — vary. At its core lies the idea that health agencies should not exist in isolation from one another and should coordinate their activities to serve the population that is their common concern. Toward this end, central government should be prepared to delegate substantial authority to some form of coordinating regional organization. The discussions at Salzburg showed varied reasons, outlined below, for the concept's appeal and a variety of structural patterns arising from it.

Sweden

In Sweden (population 8.2 million) regionalization applies largely to the hospital system, although some primary care centers are beginning. As noted in Chapter 2 there is a tidy hierarchy of district, county, and regional hospitals, and the principal management responsibility lies at the county level. Except in the big cities and the north, the population of a county is about 250,000, which is large enough to require and justify a major acute hospital. Besides receiving grants from central government, the counties have power to collect taxes, and most of their revenue (nearly 90 percent) goes to finance the hospital system. With time, the municipalities that had major hospitals have passed responsibility for them to the counties, while central government has also passed to them its management of psychiatric hospitals. The regional hospitals are run by consortia of counties, thus obviating the need for another organization level.[4]

Denmark

For Denmark (population 5.1 million), which moved toward a county system of control in 1971, the main motivation was a realization that the municipalities were too small to continue to take effective responsibility for hospitals and that variations in municipal wealth caused great variations in health services. Previously services were too fragmented to foster continuity of care or to allow flexibility of resource allocation. Again, the county size in Denmark is about 250,000.[5]

The Netherlands

The Netherlands (population 13.8 million) has been discussing regionalization for some time, and two experimental schemes have been tried. The number of regions is still in doubt, and thus far they do not seem likely to correspond to existing political entities, such as the Swedish counties. Reasons advanced include the need for closer cooperation among institutions and between hospitals and community services.

A major barrier to any tidy regionalization in the Netherlands is the heavy concentration of hospital and university resources in certain areas, especially in the west. Arguably, in a compact country, this concentration does not prevent access to services, but it does make regionalization more difficult. For the Ministry of Public

Health and Environmental Hygiene, a major attraction of regionalization is the possibility that it presents of allocating budgets on a population basis and of facing regional authorities with the task of allocating scarce resources.[6]

Greece

Greece (population 9.2 million) is currently considering regionalization for health services, probably with six to eight regions with populations from around one million to three and a half million (the Athens area). Within regions, districts already exist as administrative and political entities, with populations normally in the range of 100,000 to 150,000. Probably the districts would run the public hospitals, under regional guidance, with community health services based on health centers run by smaller local entities (population, say, 30,000). Among the main reasons for regionalization of health services in Greece is a wish to develop coherent patterns of primary, secondary, and tertiary care on a decentralized basis. A major question is how Athens should fit into such a pattern, and what part it should play as a national referral center.[7]

Ireland

In the Republic of Ireland (population 3.2 million) health services were reorganized under the Health Act of 1970. Management of all publicly administered health services passed from twenty-three counties and four urban health authorities to eight newly created Health Boards. As in Denmark, preexisting local government authorities were thought too small to plan and provide a modern health service, particularly the sophisticated, hospital element of it.

The new Health Board areas vary in size from rather less than 200,000 in the more thinly populated areas to one million in Dublin. In addition, three Regional Hospital Boards were to coordinate hospital planning, each for two or more Health Boards, but the Regional Hospital Boards have had little influence. Within the Health Boards there was emphasis on improving the quality of health administration and coordinating more closely the main branches of health services (primary care, hospitals of all kinds, services for the handicapped, and public health).

Finally, through the reorganization central government sought tighter financial control, as in the Netherlands. When the public financing of services was 50 percent from local rates, local government was keenly sensitive to increases in cost. But with central government's share becoming the dominant one, and particularly the dominant support for increases, local government ceased to exercise tight control, and a new structure was required. The Health Boards receive their budgets from the central government and are subject to central controls on expenditure.[8]

The United Kingdom

The United Kingdom (population 56 million) reorganized its health services in 1974. (England, Northern Ireland, Scotland, and Wales each has a somewhat different structure for the National Health Service.) As in the Irish Republic, the rhetoric of reorganization emphasized improved management efficiency, but in reality the case rested on the opportunity to unite interdependent services.

Up to 1974 primary care, public and community health services, general hospitals, psychiatric hospitals, and teaching hospitals were all administered by separate authorities. Since 1974, the basic organizational unit of the National Health Service in England and Wales has been the district, with a population of about 250,000 in most cases. A multidisciplinary management team is responsible for all services within the district, including teaching hospitals where appropriate. (Administration of family practitioner contracts is separate, but the liaison with family practitioner services should be close, and in many districts it is.) These district management teams are accountable to area health authorities, with boundaries corresponding in most cases to those of the local government authorities, which are responsible for social services, housing, and education.

Between the ninety area health authorities in England (but not in Wales) and central government are fourteen regional health authorities. These areas roughly correspond in size to the regional hospital boards that existed between 1948 and 1974 and have populations ranging from 1.7 million to 5.1 million. Each contains at least one medical school and major referral center. The regional health authorities and their staffs are responsible for broad strategy in their regions and particularly for medical manpower deployment, major capital construction, and the allocation of financial resources among area health authorities.

The Conservative government, elected in May 1979, proposes to simplify the overall structure. Details are not yet known, but the expectation is that areas will disappear as a separate organizational level, leaving district and regional health authorities, and a central government Department of Health.[9]

Italy

Italy (population 56 million) made major changes to the structure of its health services in January 1975. Prior to that date the structure was fragmented, each public hospital being governed by its own board, with other public medical and health services provided by several thousand municipalities, and most funding for public and private services coming from sickness insurance.

Under the new law, fifteen regions became responsible for all publicly administered hospital and health services, with funds allocated to them by the central government and drawn partly from sickness insurance and partly from general taxation. The regions, with populations varying from 100,000 to 8 million, have strong historical roots (for example, Milan, Bologna, and Venice each provides the focus for a region) and are intended to have many other functions besides health administration. Granted the background of Italian politics, the regions are likely to be strongly independent of central government.

Under the regions, local health units, usually with populations between 50,000 and 200,000 and responsible for running public hospital and health services within their boundaries, are to be created. These are new administrative entities, comprising groupings of municipalities, and are taking time to create.

The new regional structure of health services in Italy seems to have been consciously modeled on the British National Health Service, wih the aim of drawing the financing and provision of health services into an integrated whole. As remarked in Chapter 2, it is questionable if this logical structure will actually work in Italy, and still more doubtful if it will solve some of the long-standing problems of health services there.[10]

Canada

Under the British North America Act, health care in Canada (population 23 million) is the constitutional responsibility of the ten provinces. Only in the Yukon and the North West Territories does the federal government itself carry direct responsibility for health care. Federal acts of 1958 and 1966 lay down broad requirements like universality that provincial health insurance schemes must meet to qualify for federal grants, but within these guidelines provincial governments are free to choose their own schemes of funding and administration. As a result there are very substantial variations among provinces.

The populations of the provinces range from around 100,000 in Prince Edward Island to over 8 million in Ontario. In recent years there has been discussion in several provinces about forms of regionalization or of health districts. To date these new organizations are shadowy, with advisory functions only. Even in Quebec, where the Castonguay commission in 1970 recommended the establishment of three regions with wide powers, each with autonomy to provide a relatively complete range of health services for a population of at least 1 million, the regions that have actually been created as yet have little power. (They have recently been given some funds to allocate for specialized equipment and small capital projects.) There have, however, also been attempts in Quebec to strengthen the organization of community health services and to encourage hospitals to be increasingly aware of community needs and aspirations. Possibly some form of health districts will spring from this.[11]

The United States

In the United States (population 215 million) most structural questions relating to health services remain open. Only two points need to be made here. First, the differentiation of federal and state responsibilities is less clear than in Canada. Some health programs (for example, Medicaid) are largely determined by the states, even though they attract substantial federal funding, and they vary greatly in scope from one state to another. Other programs, policies and regulations are controlled in great detail centrally, despite the difficulty of doing this in so large and populous a country.

Second, there are about 200 Health Systems Agencies, created under Public Law 93-641 to plan and coordinate health services within defined geographic areas with populations ranging in some cases over the 5 million mark. By law their membership is dominated by consumers. Although their responsibilities are formidably wide ranging, their powers are chiefly advisory. In particular, state governments may, or may not, implement HSA recommendations. If they choose not to do so, the relevant HSAs would become forums solely for consultation, and for that purpose, many of them cover too large a population for all the affected parties to be represented.[12]

PROS AND CONS OF REGIONALIZATION

These examples of national developments show widespread interest in some form of regionalization of health services administration. The reasons for the interest include a wish to see health agencies coordinate their activities and relate them to public needs; an attempt to encourage flexibility in the use of limited health care resources; a bid by government to tighten expenditure control; and perhaps, an opportunity to examine and counteract disparities in the geographic distribution of health care resources.

Clearly there are national differences, not only in execution but also in perception and definition. The term regionalization has been used to describe initiatives at two different levels, one local and the other subprovincial or subnational. The local or district level requires a population of around 250,000 (less in thinly populated areas and more in urban centers), since this is the smallest population for which general hospital services can be planned sensibly. Primary care and public health activities can generally be planned for much smaller populations, but 250,000 is the least for which nearly all health care services can be planned. (The exceptions are referral specialties that may require much larger catchment populations.)

The second subprovincial or subnational level is only appropriate in provinces or countries with populations of at least 5 million. Below this level it should be possible for government to deal directly with the health authorities at local level (up to twenty of them, assuming local units of 250,000 population).

Undeniably a price has to be paid for a reorganization that creates local, district units of administration and (when appropriate) subprovincial or subnational groupings of these local units. The price includes the confusion, inefficiency, and demoralization noted by Petronius. It also includes some erosion of the independence and traditions of existing institutions, with the loyalty and cooperation engendered by them. Institutional strength takes a long time to build. Inevitably it creates a district administrative level more remote from the workplace because it is responsible for a range of services, not for a single institution. Staff properly miss the intimacy of contact with board and management to which they were accustomed. And (particularly where a subprovincial or subnational level is also required) communication between each institution and the government is hampered by the interpolation of new organizational layers. Finally, there is a serious danger that when the new district organizations have taken root, they will become isolationist in seeking to be self-sufficient in the provision of services and to discourage the movement of patients across administrative boundaries. Apart from diminishing freedom of choice, this tendency ignores the vital need for referral centers and for not duplicating in every district activities that should be concentrated in such centers.

Taking all these factors into the balance, the price of regionalization is a heavy one. Nevertheless, it is worth paying to create a coordinated health service that is planned and provided for a specific population. Using the assessment criteria with which this chapter opened, a district-based organization seems to me markedly superior to any other for the purposes of relating health services to needs and for using limited health care resources to best effect. It should also be possible to meet the other criteria — acceptability and suitability, simplicity and comprehensibility, and cost.

OTHER ISSUES

Assuming that regionalization (particularly the creation of health districts) is accepted in principle, there are consequential questions about the range of services to be included; the appropriate membership and method of election or appointment of the new authorities; and the clear definition of the roles, functions, and powers of the various organizational bodies that need to work together, their staffing, and their working methods and procedures, including the ways in which they will receive funds, allocate them, and control expenditure. To most of these questions there is no one right answer. The best answer will depend, among other things, on a sense of what is acceptable and appropriate in the particular social context. In general, however, a large measure of decentralization from government to the local level is fundamental.

People locally — public and staff — must know the rules and resource limits within which agencies are to provide the best care they can. And they must have responsibility for taking decisions on priorities and power to implement these decisions. Decentralization to regions and to districts on this basis is bound to lead to mistakes, some of them embarrassing. But even if greater centralization would avoid mistakes, which I doubt, local initiative is to be preferred because health care has to be responsive to needs and opportunities that vary substantially from place to place and because choices posed by limited health care resources cannot all be made centrally.

NOTES

1. Petronius, *The Satyricon,* A.D. 66.
2. Wilfred Brown, *Exploration in Management* (London: Heinemann, 1960; Pelican Books, 1965).
3. Sir Harold Himsworth, *The Development and Organisation of Scientific Knowledge* (London: Heinemann, 1970).

4. See V. Navarro, *National and Regional Health Planning in Sweden* (Washington, D.C.: Fogarty Center, DHEW, 1974). For other references about health care in Sweden, see Chapter 1.
5. See D. Gannik, E. Holst, and M. Wagner, *The National Health System in Denmark* (Washington, D.C.: Fogarty Center, DHEW, 1976).
6. For background reading on health services in the Netherlands, see Chapter 1. Regionalization was proposed in about 1975 when J. P. M. Hendriks was secretary of state for health and the environment in the Netherlands. Memoranda from the ministry were widely circulated at the time, and two experimental schemes were launched.
7. So far as I am aware, nothing has yet been published in English about proposals for regionalization of health services in Greece.
8. See B. Hersey, *The Health Services of Ireland* (Dublin: Institute of Public Administration, 1972).
9. See R. Levitt, *The Reorganised National Health Service* (London: Croom Helm, 1976).
10. See A. Maynard, *Health Care in the European Community* (London: Croom Helm, 1975), ch. 7.
11. For Canada generally see P. Soderstrom, *The Canadian Health System* (London: Croom Helm Ltd., 1977). For Quebec see S. S. Lee, *Quebec's Health System: A Decade of Change, 1967-77*, Monographs on Canadian Public Administration No. 4 (The Institute of Public Administration of Canada, 1979).
12. On HSAs and PL 93-641 see S. Sieverts, *Health Planning Issues and Public Law 93-641* (Chicago: American Hospital Association, 1977).

Chapter 8

The Organization of Primary Care in Israel

Haim R. Doron, M.D.
in collaboration with Aviva Ron

INTRODUCTION

The network of primary health care delivery in Israel was first established by the pioneers in agricultural settlement at the beginning of the century. Their guiding objectives were to combat physical difficulties, to build a new way of life that suited their ideals of social and national redemption, and at the same time to mold a society based on equality and mutual aid. In this environment, these settlers had to surmount innumerable difficulties, including endemic infectious diseases, making their health care a daily struggle. A special kind of relationship therefore evolved between the physician-nurse team and the settler patient. In most cases, the physician and nurse were part of the same group of initiators of the new social structure and blended these ideals with their professional realization. The physician, the nurse, and the patient were very often members of the same kibbutz or cooperative farm, sharing an indomitable will to survive in a well-established and defendable settlement.

The resulting warm and friendly doctor-patient relationship, full of personal as well as social concern, was the cornerstone of a widespread network of health services based on health insurance sponsored by the Sick Fund of the General Federation of Labour in Israel, henceforth called Kupat Holim. This health services system provides comprehensive health care for an insured population of 2.9 million, or 77 percent of Israel's total population in 1979. These are members of the Labour Federation and their dependents, including retired parents over sixty-five years of age. In addition, Kupat Holim insures self-employed individuals, regardless of union membership, and their dependents. Health services are also provided for over 100,000 welfare recipients through a global agreement with the Ministry of Labour and Social Affairs. It should be noted that an additional 20 percent of the population are insured by four other small sick funds.

A very important aspect of the system is that Kupat Holim not only provides health insurance but also builds, owns, and operates care facilities, employing physicians; nurses; and paramedical, administrative, teaching and research staff as full-time salaried employees. Kupat Holim owns approximately one-third of the general hospital beds in eight hospitals in various parts of the country. In areas where Kupat Holim has no hospital, services (inpatient as well as casualty and outpatient consultation) are purchased from government or voluntary hospitals in that area, at the charge fixed by the government. In other areas, where Kupat Holim does operate a hospital facility, services are provided to non-Kupat Holim members at the same charge. Ambulatory physician and ancillary services are provided in 1400 clinics in all parts of the country, with primary care clinics located in each community or settlement. In areas where Kupat Holim operates a general hospital, specialist services are integrated with the hospital services and are usually located in the outpatient department. In areas where Kupat Holim relies on other agencies for hospital care, specialty clinics have been developed in urban centers to serve the district population. These specialty clinics rely on referral to the local hospital for inpatient care, regardless of hospital ownership. Routine laboratory and X-ray diagnostic services are generally provided in the ambulatory facilities, on a district basis.

In addition to the general hospitals, Kupat Holim operates four long-term rehabilitation and chronic disease hospitals and four psychiatric institutions. Both types of special hospitals have inpatient, day care, and consultation units, employing a broad range of medical, nursing, social, and vocational services. Additional facilities serving the insured population are a network of convalescent homes, most of which are located in resort areas of the country. In recent years dental clinics have been established, although dental care is currently not covered by the insurance. Dental services are provided to Kupat Holim members in dental clinics owned and operated by Kupat Holim at rates considerably lower than current private prices. Kupat Holim is extensively involved in undergraduate and postgraduate training of medical and paramedical personnel, using both community and hospital facilities for teaching. Research is carried out in clinical, biomedical, and social science fields, generally in affiliation with the country's universities and scientific institutions.

Following this brief description of the foundation of the Kupat Holim primary care network and the general context of the institution, this chapter will deal with the basic concepts of primary care, its loci and providers, new functions, relationships with other services, education for primary care, and the information system required.

The Kupat Holim primary care network has been developed on the basis of some of the fundamental principles expounded by Dr. Joseph Meir (1890-1953)[1]:

1. A high level of medical care.
2. The nondependence of the doctor-patient relationship on the ability of the patient to pay fees.
3. A concern for family health, not just for the individual.
4. Coverage of all health care stages — prevention, treatment, and rehabilitation — with due attention to continuity of care and coordination between the three stages.

The expansion of this form of health insurance in Israel brought in its wake the development of health care facilities in every corner of the country, in villages or agricultural settlements without regard to size. This process included the development of community and hospital services, mental health, rehabilitation, and general nursing care both in the community and in hospitals. Such expansion and diversity of the services necessitated a well-organized administration and delivery patterns to fit the current needs, while reflecting the basic concepts of the health care system. The fundamental directives in this concept are the designation of a community health team as the front line provider of care on the one hand and as the coordinators of all health interests pertaining to the individual member and his or her family on the other.

This development of public health services without the parallel development of private medical practice on the same scale during these years was also influenced by the nature of current physician manpower — primarily new immigrant physicians coming from different countries and various medical schools. Because of the professional backgrounds of these new immigrant physicians, a great number of them had to be retrained from hospital-based specialties to general medicine or given posts in a broad range of specialties in community and district clinics in order to be absorbed into the system. Neither the providers nor the patients could afford a private entrepreneurial health care system and sought the facilities, stability, and comprehensiveness provided by Kupat Holim in a developing economy and society.

The changes that have taken place in the disease pattern and morbidity in the last several decades have placed community disease — heart disease, cancer, and stroke — at the head of the list of main causes of illness and death among adults in the society. The nature of these diseases and the factors related to their etiology have strengthened the rationale of the basic concepts of this health care system, specifically the integration of health promotion into preventive medicine, curative medicine, and rehabilitation. This concept also does not separate organic or physical factors from the mental health aspects, all of which are seen in a broad medicosocial spectrum.

THE LOCUS OF PRIMARY CARE SERVICES

The locus of activity of the providers of primary care can be classified as follows:

1. The community clinic (urban or rural);
2. The clinic of the physician in his home;
3. The patient's home;
4. The patient's place of work;
5. At school or in educational institutions.

Primary care services in the Kupat Holim framework have principally been developed in community clinics. This development first occurred in agricultural settlements, in kibbutzim or cooperatives, and was later shaped by the urban society of the new immigrants. As a result of this situation and as the majority of the insured were new immigrants, including most physicians, nurses, and other workers, the development of the community clinic became not only the cornerstone of the system of health care services and the center of primary health care, but also the foundation of the new social structure by which we can understand the complexity of the socialization process of new immigrants. In the course of time, the clinics have undergone different variations in size, structure, function, and scope of activities.

The rural unit, which is the smallest clinic, basically consists of doctor's room, nurse's room, a small drug dispensary, treatment room, waiting room, and in many cases, a dental clinic. In many of these rural clinics, personal preventive care is provided, with maternal and child care being given in the same framework, whereas elsewhere, curative services and preventive medicine are often completely separate, the latter provided by local authorities under Ministry of Health auspices. With the conviction that curative services and preventive medicine should be combined, rural health centers have been developed in recent years in which integrated health care is provided for a number of rural settlements. While most care is given in the health center, each settlement maintains a nurse station, and the physician makes home calls when necessary. Such a rural health center generally provides care for a total of several thousand residents in a number of settlements with a radius of no more than 7 to 10 kilometers. The urban clinics differ in size according to the needs of the populations under their care. The family practitioner's list has 1400 patients on average, and the pediatrician's 1000 children. An urban community clinic consists of doctors' rooms, nurses' rooms, a pharmacy, office, and waiting room. Some urban clinics include consulting rooms for specialists, mainly for gynecology-obstetrics, and some have a laboratory for routine tests and serve an average population of 10,000 residents.

For many years, there was a distinct separation between doctors' rooms and the nurses' treatment room. During the past fifteen years, the need to expand the nurse's role in medical functions, including social and rehabilitation tasks, gave rise to a new concept of health care delivery in these clinics by introducing a physician-nurse team. The participation of the nurse in preparing the patient's first visit to the physician and maintaining later contacts requires certain changes in clinic design to allow enough space for the various functions. The layout must permit physician-nurse team work, health education activities, and consultations with other health care workers such as dietitians or social workers and must allow for staff conferences.

The astounding development of family medicine and primary health care in medical schools, the expanded specialization programs in these disciplines, and the resulting establishment of the accredited units for teaching and specialization also require adequate space allocation. The primary community clinic unit consisting principally of consultation rooms for the physicians and treatment rooms for the nurses has gradually changed into a clinic team unit with medical secretaries. This concept has grown into teaching clinics, which could serve as centers for services and research in health and community health care. This community unit forms the foundation for health promotion, prevention of disease, treatment, and rehabilitation and will increasingly integrate the delivery of health care, teaching, and research carried out by multidisciplinary professionals.

One may ask if such an institution answers the needs for more privacy in the physician-patient relationship. This question is particularly hard put with regard to neighborhoods and areas with more complex social characteristics, densely populated with new immigrants, and with an abundance of medicosocial problems. With the improvement in the standard of living, people demand more consultations in the privacy of the physician's home. A trial system termed "independent physician" was initiated several years ago by Kupat Holim as a complementary system to the primary community clinic and at the free choice of the member. This complementary system enables the member to be seen in the home of the physician, who is paid on a per capita basis by the institution and not directly by the patient. It is worth mentioning that despite the fact that some dissatisfaction is felt regarding the clinic services, the parallel system in the physician's home has not brought about a sharp decrease in the affiliation with the clinics. Plausible reasons may be that all the various services are concentrated in the same building or that conservative habits are stronger than new trends. The "independent physician" who receives patients in his home has not significantly attracted members from the primary community clinic in Israel, which has retained its central strength and increased in function.

So far, we have dealt with primary health care within the public system. There is, as well, private medicine in Israel, and it has expanded considerably during the past few years, but has generally remained confined to specific fields and does not upset the stability of the public primary community health care system. The view that has developed regarding the content and scope of primary community health care tends to see a physician-patient contact in the physician's home as a single episode within the spectrum of the multiprofessional activities of primary community health care delivery. With due importance to the nature of the physician-patient relationship in the different milieu, each contact should be an integral part of the individual's care, particularly when at the primary care level. The structure of the community clinic as it has developed at the local level and with a team of health and related professionals seems the right response to this issue.

We attach much importance to the inclusion of the patient's home in the loci of activities of primary health care. Increasingly frequent are the followup home visits initiated by clinic nurses to patients with chronic diseases, and the nursing and rehabilitation activities of the multiprofessional community teams within the framework of district home care units complement the system's activities in the member's home.

The development of occupational health services is considered an important part of Kupat Holim services, with the provision of services for workers in large and specific enterprises. These services are oriented toward preventive medicine and the monitoring of risks of a particular occupation. At the same time, we have to take care not to create a duplicate system of curative services parallel or in addition to primary medical care in the community. This remark, of course, does not apply to the indispensable elements of first aid. The same caution against duplication holds true with regard to personal preventive health care provided in schools. Primary health care delivered to students on the premises of higher educational establishments, however, is of a different nature, which we will not describe in this framework.

THE PROVIDERS OF PRIMARY HEALTH CARE

The subject of general practitioner versus family doctor, or primary internist and primary pediatrician in the front line team, is at the center of discussions and debates in health organizations all over the world. On our part, we have developed both patterns, but in recent years, emphasis has been placed on the pattern in which the family doctor is responsible for the health of the whole family with all its components and encompasses basic preventive and psychosocial aspects in his or her diagnostic and treatment activities. The education of this physician is one of the goals of the family medicine units that have been established in medical schools in Israel.

Training for this framework of family practice takes place not only in the medical school but from a very early stage at the residency level, in the primary care community clinic described above. Kupat Holim has taken upon itself responsibility for finding residency posts in family medicine for young doctors in its community clinics and hospitals. The Scientific Council of the Israel Medical Association has agreed to a specialization syllabus of four and a half years that has been authorized by the Israel Ministry of Health. Half of this period is devoted to rotation in hospitals, and the other half is supervised practice in family health clinics in the community. Academic courses in community medicine and family medicine in the university and clinic setting complete the training of the young doctor destined to this post. The basic intention is to bring about changes in the specialization trends of medical graduates in order to curtail the tide to hospital-based specialties and direct them to family and community medicine.

An additional significant development is the establishment of a Medical School in the Negev, in the south of Israel. This is a joint venture of the Kupat Holim Health Insurance Institution and the Faculty of Medical Sciences of the Ben-Gurion University, thereby combining under the same authority the delivery of services, training, and research. The major objective of this endeavor is to educate a different kind of doctor, who will find his or her principal occupation and interest in community and primary health care. To implement this mission, many changes have had to be made, beginning with the system of selection of applicants in order to accept those with the most suitable motivation and background and the compilation of a new curriculum with orientation toward family and community practice as opposed to the classical methods of teaching medicine.

Those who favor primary internal medicine emphasize the central role of internal medicine in the formation of the doctor and his or her practice, while the promoters of family medicine will stress the necessity of basic knowledge in more specific medical branches, such as mental health, and medicosocial aspects. Another difference lies in the division of the family between adults under the primary internist and children under primary pediatric care, while the family doctor will treat the whole family. In our opinion, if there is no contradiction between the knowledge necessary for the fulfillment of primary health care and its real essence, these differences will remain controversial, and the implementation of this goal will be attained when the appropriate organization, manpower, and the consumer requirements will be met.

We must bear in mind that the development of primary health care cannot be solely based on the doctor's work. The range of services in current concepts of primary care should be provided by a team with the doctor at its head, and with nurses, social workers, pharmacists, laboratory technicians, medical secretaries, and additional ancillary health services. The common scientific training of these team members must include epidemiology and biostatistics, behavioral sciences, and the principles of public health — all with a background of solid and updated medical knowledge. The basic team in the Kupat Holim community clinics was formed when a nurse was added to the primary doctor. The classical training of the nurse hardly provides a grounding to suit the new health care and social functions. Our present aim is to train nurses in community health care, on the premise that this training will not only be beneficial to the family and community health unit, but will also permit the doctor to devote more time to clinical functions, education, and research.

NEW FUNCTIONS OF THE PRIMARY CARE TEAM

Over the past decade we have increasingly added the terms health education, health promotion, and more recently, "self-care" to the medical care lexicon. While these are in fact very old forms of health care, their reintroduction has implications primarily for the primary care team. This team has become not only the front line provider, with continuous responsibility for the individual's health, but also the closest and most frequent observer of the individual patient's health and lifestyle. It is not enough to designate responsibility for these new functions to the primary care team. Effective health education requires knowledge in behavioral sciences and communication, apart from being up to date in the epidemiology and etiology of current diseases. Above all, effective health education requires a sound noncoercive provider-patient relationship, based on mutual respect.

Since we see the Kupat Holim primary care community clinics as a suitable milieu for health education, considerable efforts have been made to formalize these new functions. Health education is now considered an integral part of daily practice, after the primary care teams undergo appropriate training, and reinforcement is provided by central and district health educators. The prime issues dealt with today are the changes in habits and lifestyle related to preventing illness, early detection of illness, and effective and appropriate treatment at all stages of care. This requires active awareness of the population at risk, identification of early stages of disease, and harnessing the appropriate treatment and medical care tools for all stages, both within the community clinic and beyond. The teams are taught that health education is to be provided not only to the "community" at large but primarily to the individual patient with whom the direct and ongoing relationship exists.

THE RELATIONSHIP BETWEEN PRIMARY CARE AND OTHER HEALTH SERVICES

The relationship between the primary team and the specialty services is based on two main factors: (1) the composition of the primary team in terms of its professional qualifications in each particular branch of primary care; and (2) the composition of specialists services and their integration with hospitals. It is clear that the presence of a pediatrician in the primary clinic will certainly enable extension of the scope of work in prevention and treatment and thereby diminish referrals for additional pediatric consultation. The same applies when a gynecologist is added to the primary health team.

Over many years, a three-tiered structure had developed in which the insured member is referred from the primary care clinic to a consultant in the district or regional clinic. The cases that needed further diagnosis or special treatment in hospitals were referred to the third station — the hospital. The development of this structure is partially due to the absorption of new immigrant physicians, who included a very high proportion of specialists. In recent years, however, two patterns were promoted to improve the overall level of ambulatory specialty services: (1) the expansion of hospital outpatient departments not only for followup, but also to provide direct consultation to the primary doctor; and (2) referral of specialists from hospitals to the primary care clinics for consultation in the community. This process transforms the three-tiered structure to a two-tiered system and greatly contributes to the improvement of the primary care level, which benefits from on the spot counseling.

To implement the system, two additional organizational changes were made. First, specific primary care clinics were linked to defined hospital departments in the designated regional hospital. Second, all Kupat Holim hospital duty rosters changed to accept casualties and admissions on a daily basis each day of the week. Previously, this duty had been split between two or more hospitals during the week, so that a patient might well be hospitalized in a different hospital when readmission was necessary.

The next stage in this process deals with integration of work between primary clinic and hospital. There is a school of thought that sponsors the noncompatibility aspects between the two functions, and while admitting the difficulties on this subject, we do not entirely agree with an absolute total noncompatibility structure. The combination of practice in the community and in hospital is more feasible in pediatrics and with rural physicians working in settlements in the vicinity of the district hospitals. This combination, though rather complicated, is extremely difficult to implement in urban family medicine. The "closed" Israeli hospital, which resembles the British pattern in staff structure, contributes to this difficulty. This structure does not allow the easy integration of the same doctor between the community and the hospital.

In addition to these links with general acute hospital services, the primary care team has developed an on-going relationship with long-term and rehabilitation services. There must be close contact between the community health system and medical and occupational rehabilitation services either in the community or in institutions. The primary care team's aim is to help insure the reintegration of the patient to normal life within his or her family, work, and community.

EDUCATION FOR PRIMARY CARE

The trend toward creating a renaissance in primary medicine requires parallel change in two basic fields — medical education and the delivery of services. Partial changes in services or education alone will not help obtain far-reaching compensations to assure the expansion of health care services and improvement in its quality or to attract young and professional manpower to join the ranks of primary care. The changes in medical education brought about by the establishment of the Faculty of Medical Sciences in the Negev region described above and the development of family medicine and primary medicine units in all the country's medical schools are linked to the development of accredited tuition clinics. In these clinics the multidisciplinary teams have been expanded, beginning with the dotor-nurse team and a list of members that enables the statistical followup of groups of patients with selected diseases. Regular staff meetings take place relating to professional and organizational subjects, and many activities are carried out. The clinics have been renovated, and equipment has been added to further tuition objectives.

Currently, the training of teachers and supervisors, particularly in these clinics, is a central issue in the specialization programs. Regular programs of postgraduate medical education for primary physicians have also been organized and expanded over the years. The aim is not only to update clinical knowledge, but also to provide a continuous link between primary physicians and the regional hospital. These programs have several forms, the principal one being a fixed day each week that the primary physicians spend in hospitals, particularly in the department hospitalizing their patients, and under the guidance of senior physicians of the same institution. This fixed study day is a professional privilege that also entails defined obligations. Individual training programs for primary physicians in regional hospitals and courses on specific subjects complement the study programs.

These programs, however, are only a first step in the process of integration of the primary physician with the regional hospital. The physician who perseveres in training activities, receives an "affiliated physician" status, which designates a specific function in the regional hospital to which his or her clinic is attached and in which hospital he or she performs these duties for several hours a week. In this program, special reference is made to the retraining of new immigrant physicians. In view of their varied origins and medical backgrounds, they must undergo special training to enable them to fulfill their new functions adequately and to acquaint them with the functioning of the health system in their new surroundings.

The programs have two basic directions — first, to increase diagnostic and therapeutic knowledge, and second, to broaden their concepts of preventive medicine, health promotion, rehabilitation, nursing care, mental health, health insurance, and the medicosocial problems in the community. These two directions do not conflict with each other; on the contrary, they are complementary in the training program. The latter direction is aimed at changing and broadening the knowledge and attitudes of the community physician educated in the classical school, with its clinical and curative medicine emphasis. For this purpose, among the many activities undertaken for the development of community medicine, two-year courses have been introduced with a curriculum including epidemiology, principles of public health, behavioral sciences, biostatistics, and the organization of medical care.

To complement all the above, and to deal with changes in the age structure and related morbidity pattern of the population, chronic disease control training has been added in the last several years. In this program, specialist teams systematically train community clinic doctors and nurses in early detection and followup care of patients with chronic diseases. This training emphasizes not only the current knowledge on the etiology and epidemiology of the major chronic diseases, but brings to the primary care team updated clinical and pharmacological knowledge.

THE PRIMARY CARE INFORMATION SYSTEM

The primary care information system must answer a broad range of needs, the scope depending on the overall system of care. In all health care systems, from private solo practice to group practice in publicly owned community clinics, the information set must first focus on the individual within a family. As the system claims greater accountability and responsibility for community health, the primary care information set must serve the needs for records of services provided to the community, with focus on the content of practice. This content must include epidemiological as well as resource utilization information. A basic requirement of primary care records is that they enable evaluation of quality of care, both that given to the patient and that given to the community or clinic population. In any health care system, the content of practice records, such as the daily or monthly clinic diaries, should not be emphasized at the expense of the individual patient record. Whereas population information can always be extracted from events recorded for individuals in their own files, the incomplete and inadequately filled patient record reflects defective patient care.

To these requirements we must add another dimension. Primary care is no longer provided only by physicians, but by nurses too — and increasingly by a team comprising doctors, nurses, dietitians, pharmacists, social workers, and others. At the same time, primary care is no longer strictly medical care given to the individual, but now includes related services given to the individual and his family members, sometimes involving educational, welfare, or occupational agencies. This means that the information set must allow for continuity of care by the physician on the one hand and relevant team access on the other, while at the same time safeguarding the patient's medicolegal rights to secrecy. A multidisciplinary range of providers, automated information systems, and sophisticated and seemingly impersonal data storage and retrieval systems may indeed constitute positive changes in modern health care, yet they should in no way jeopardize the basic rights of the individual for both personal health care and discretion.

Requirements for the clarity of forms, brevity, and compactness, as well as record accessibility, have become accepted as necessary attributes in developing primary care information systems. Focus on the expansion of these systems in the last decade has been placed more on the uses of information in primary family practice. Clinical management is generally listed first, with practice management or content study second. As an important by-product, the total primary care record set should serve as a data source for research in primary care, thereby increasing the need for completeness and accuracy in recording. Trials with the problem-oriented record introduced by Weed were aimed at serving mainly the first uses — that is, clinical management. The use of computers in family practice is promoted more by the needs of data linkage in complex health services systems, the acceptance of the comprehensiveness of medical care, and the more general applications of computers in medicine.

To all the above, we must add an appropriate sense of proportion, in terms of the number of forms and charts; the time required by the medical staff to complete these forms accurately; and the clerical staff needed to set up and maintain the various record systems, registries, and ledgers. As primary care moves to group and team patterns, with area health centers serving the needs of several small communities, it may well be that the economies of scale thereby achieved will allow for more clerical positions. Yet these changes in delivery patterns are often made in times of economic constraint, so that the addition of new kinds of personnel to deal with paperwork does not generally receive the well-calculated consideration it may deserve. In an atmosphere of scarce resources, the choice between a secretary or an additional nurse in the primary care clinic is difficult to make, even when job analysis shows that the nurse spends a considerable proportion of her time carrying out clerical tasks.

The information system currently used in the Kupat Holim primary care clinics does not answer all the needs described above, mainly because its primary care community clinic system is so much older and broader than the primary care information systems developed over the last two decades at most. Implementing new concepts in a network of some 1400 clinics throughout the country, served by some 5000 doctors and nurses, obviously entails more problems than these encountered in changing medical records in a single self-motivated practice. Resistance to change is not only multiplied, but must also be dealt with by different methods when dealing with doctors who have come from different medical educational backgrounds and who have worked within the system for varying lengths of time. The current information system is a mixture of old and new in which such new concepts as family care, monitoring of the patient with chronic diseases, problem recording, patient load, and referrals have been introduced into the basic record system. Most of these changes occurred in the last fifteen years, and it is important to stress that the changes were implemented when decisions of the Kupat Holim Central Executive reflected initiative of a group of direct providers of care (doctors and nurses working in the community clinics) or at least gained support of the clinic staff. New tools were therefore not imposed on the primary care network but introduced gradually, usually following pilot stages with voluntary participation of selected clinics.

Only the major elements of this system are described here, as it would be superfluous and irrelevant to describe every form, register, and legend found in the large community clinic network of a complex and necessarily bureaucratic health care system. The elements described relate to the individual patient record, the direct provider (doctor and nurse) record, and the relevant general clinic registries.

The Patient Record

The individual record is a loose-leaf folder, the contents of which have changed significantly over time. Originally, the folder was designed to hold "contact sheets," on which the date, reason, and content of each patient visit to the clinic doctor were recorded. The folder was designed with a pocket for the filing of results of tests (such as laboratory and X-ray) as well as hospital discharge summaries. Currently, the folder has three basic types of sheets:

a summary page, on which past and current problems are listed, with additional separate spaces for risk factors, family illnesses, hospitalizations, and referrals;
current visit sheets, on which reasons for visit and content are recorded; and
chronic-disease-monitoring sheets, where a range of parameters specific to selected chronic diseases are recorded over time, allowing appraisal of the disease process in the individual. Such sheets have been developed for hypertension, diabetes, and other diseases.

Long before the worldwide trend toward family medicine, the individual patient records were filed with those of other family members, in a family folder. In clinics where pediatricians provide primary care of children, the younger members of the family have their own "family" folder.

The Provider Record

Since the initial development of Kupat Holim community clinics, the physicians have filled in a daily diary of clinic and home visits on which the patient's name, sex, age, diagnosis, and type of visit (first, repeat, home) were recorded. These daily diaries were used to abstract morbidity data for the monthly returns set to the Central Executive and to the Ministry of Health for the reporting of notifiable diseases. In clinics where doctor-nurse teamwork was introduced, the nurse filled in a similar diary, with emphasis on the recording of content of the visit (such as blood pressure measurement and insulin administration). A major and very significant change in the physician diary was implemented in this last year. Following several pilot surveys in different parts of the country and of different physician groups, the daily diary was changed to a log sheet allowing recording of the content of the visit as well as the previously noted data. Content includes note of drug prescription, referrals for laboratory and X-ray services, and referrals to specialists and hospital services. Another change was in the heading of the "reason" column, where symptoms have been added to diagnosis. This record is precoded for analysis by computer and obviously serves as an excellent tool for the study of a wide range of parameters, from clinic load to ambulatory morbidity patterns to drug prescribing and referral dates.

The Clinic Registry

In a health insurance system in which membership is based on the regular monthly payment of dues, a complete and updated membership file is essential. A by-product of such a file is the production of lists or registries that can be used as service denominators. Developed over the past decade, alphabetical computer printouts of all individuals within families are distributed to each clinic and include basic demographic data as well as the physician under whose care the patient is listed. These lists are updated quarterly, and statistical analyses, such as the age distribution of a physician's list or total clinic list, are available on request from the Central Executive. This basic register, therefore, forms an essential element in the analysis of clinic practice and in future planning.

If this chapter were being written a decade from now, it would probably make more frequent use of words such as computer terminals, linkage, storage and retrieval, and so on. Our system has not widely promoted computerization of the primary care clinic record to date. Experiences with the computerization of primary care information in other systems and countries do not yet provide adequate analysis and guidance for its broad implementation. The major emphasis in our development has been related to our general concern for complete and accurate recording by all providers, covering not only all the relevant events but also allowing for the introduction of changes in the records to deal with changing primary care practice. This task is never completed, yet the progress made to date should allow greater consideration of new technologies, including direct use of the computer. In this future stage, emphasis must be given to remembering the patient as the principal in the information system and to considering whether the new tools developed will serve to expand and link data on the patient or reflect the quality of care provided in the primary care setting.

THE RELATIONSHIP BETWEEN PRIMARY HEALTH CARE AND OTHER COMMUNITY SERVICES

The acceptance by society of the changing components of the concept of health has led to a multiplicity of agencies dealing with the various aspects of health care. We find these other service agencies in government institutions in which health care is viewed as contributing to general welfare, such as functional and vocational rehabilitation. We find academic institutions dealing with the training of health workers and with the study of clinical and behavioral aspects of health. In recent years we find industrial agencies concerned with health, and this concern may be motivated by concern over the welfare of workers or even the marketing of their products. Then there are very specific agencies, developed initially by philanthropic and voluntary organizations, dealing with the needs of such groups as the mentally handicapped, deaf-mutes, cancer patients, and others, where often the health care component is of primary importance in the functioning of the individual. If we appraise the current situation, we find a wide range of organizations dealing with aspects of health care, with the medical institutions at one end of the spectrum; social, educational, and labor organizations in the center; and possibly industrial concerns at the other end. Rather than outright duplication of services, we hear more about individuals "falling between the seats." There may in fact be duplication of several stages or kinds of services, particularly in the diagnostic sphere, but a lack of continuity prevails, especially in the areas of medical and vocational rehabilitation.

Along with the trend to expand the spectrum of medical care, the costs of providing health and welfare services have risen drastically. Duplication has simply become too expensive, particularly for public agencies. Another factor is the shortage of competent manpower in the sociomedical fields. Specially trained social workers are in short supply, as are the newer types of professionals dealing with, for example, relevant functional assessment and vocational retraining and job placement after work and road accidents. This manpower shortage makes coordination between health and other agencies crucial in providing the effective comprehensive care we are all striving for.

The relationship between primary care and other community services within the Kupat Holim network reflects mainly the emphasis on coordination and the avoidance of duplication. Although Kupat Holim of the General Federation of Labour does not cover the entire population, it is spread all over the country and is accepted as the major provider of health care in the community. This status has become a tradition, as Kupat Holim and, in particular, its primary care elements, have existed for many years, even before the establishment of the state of Israel. This process has led to strong ties between Kupat Holim services and educational, social, labor, and other services, at all levels. While the general policies of cooperation may be set at the national level, it is in fact at the community level that these policies are most manifest.

NOTE

1. Dr. Joseph Meir, *Medicine and the Public* (Tel Aviv, 1955).

REFERENCES

Boufford, J. I. "Primary Care Residency Training: The First Five Years." *Annals of Internal Medicine* 87, No. 3 (September 1977): 359-368.

Brody, B. L., and J. Stokes III. "The Importance of Heart Disease, Cancer and Stroke in the Community Practice of Medicine." *American Journal of Public Health* (February 1972): 181-185.

Deuschle, K. W., and S. J. Bosch. "Primary Care and Community Medicine." *The Mount Sinai Journal of Medicine* 44, No. 5 (September-October 1977): 639-644.

Doron, H., and A. Ron. "Physician Integration." *Kupat Holim Yearbook*, Vol. 2 (1973), pp. 9-24.

Harding, W. G. "Community Medicine—Now." *Community Medicine* 126, No. 1 (July 2, 1971): 5-6.

Larkins, N. "The Patient, the Hospital and the General Practitioner in the 1970's." *Medical Journal of Australia* 1 (1971): 885-888.

Linden, V. "Consumers' and Doctors' View of Social Services." *Acta Socio-Medica Scandinavia* 1 (1971): 125-140.

McEwin, R., and W. S. Lawson. "The Communication Gap between Hospital and Family Doctor." *The Medical Journal of Australia* (June 19, 1971): 1334-1339.

McFarlane, A. H., G. R. Norman, and W. O. Spitzer. "Family Medicine: The Dilemma of Defining the Discipline." *C.M.A. Journal* 105 (August 21, 1971): 397-401.

Pierson, S., J. K. Glenn, and R. W. Hofmeister. "Some Considerations in the Design of Family Practice Residency Experiences." *Journal of Medical Education* 52 (July 1977): 555-561.

Polliak, M. R., and P. H. Sive. *Specialisation in Family Medicine.* Israel Medical Association. Tel Aviv: The Family Physician, Kupat Holim Health Insurance Institution, 1978, pp. 3-19.

Stoeckle, J. D., and L. M. Candib. "The Neighborhood Health Center—Reform Ideas of Yesterday and Today." *The New England Journal of Medicine* 280 (June 19, 1969): 1385-1391.

Vanderwoort, H. E., and D. C. Ransom. "A Basic Course in Family Medicine." *Journal of Medical Education* 47 (November 1972): 908-909.

Warren, M. D. "Medical Records in Family Practice." *Scandinavian Journal of Social Medicine* 4 (1976): 91-101.

West, S. R. "The Continuing Education Needs of General Practitioners." *New Zealand Medical Journal* 84, No. 572 (September 22, 1976): 225-229.

Wolfe, S., and R. F. Badgley. "The Family Doctor 1960 to 2000 A.D." *Medical Care* 11, No. 5 (September-October 1973).

Chapter 9

Consumer Participation in Formulating Health Policy

Herbert P. Gleason

In Chapter 8, Dr. Doron describes the primary health care mechanism in Israel. He portrays it as an integral part of a coherent system — the convenient entry point where a person's complaint is addressed swiftly and appropriately. From that point, necessary referrals are made to higher technological levels of the system.

No parallel can be drawn with what happens in the United States. Here, there is no established way of entering the system. Local primary facilities are often missing, so that people with minor complaints address themselves to the emergency wards of general hospitals, where their care is often delayed, inappropriate, and expensive. They may even be admitted as inpatients, because they have no access to a facility where treatment can be provided on an ambulatory basis.

Until now our national affluence has allowed providers in the United States to offer the highest technology treatment for every complaint. But as more and more people have demanded the same level of care, costs have exploded; the annual rate of increase in 1977 was 12 percent, while the consumer price index rose 10.2 percent. Expenditures for health care accounted for 8.8 percent of the gross national product or $163 billion.[1]

Alarm at the escalation in health care costs has produced proposals for caps on costs throughout the system, particularly with respect to hospitals, which in 1977 consumed 40 percent of total medical expenditures. But so long as people regard the most expensive care as the best, caps on expenditures are not going to hold.[2] They are denounced by idealists and vested interests alike as inequitable if not inhumane. The demand can only be met at less drastic cost in more simple and accessible facilities than general hospitals.

This obvious truth is finally gaining adherents in the United States, and none too soon, for there is a danger that primary care facilities, such as neighborhood health centers, are the most likely victims of the nation's decision not to allocate any larger share of resources to the health area. They are small and hence less politically effective than hospitals each of which employs thousands of unionized employees, buys from hundreds of suppliers, and is run by scores of influential trustees and professionals.[3] Moreover, because our reimbursement system favors inpatient care, ambulatory facilities are always on the verge of insolvency, requiring special public subvention. And providing wider geographical and professional services of course looks like an add-on to already strained budgets.

Fortunately in Boston there already exists a network of neighborhood health centers. In 1969, the city government inaugurated a program to strengthen or initiate local health centers throughout the city in response to a demand for medical care which was rising at the same time that private physicians were vanishing from the city's neighborhoods. The community reacted enthusiastically, and there are now twenty-six neighborhood health centers, each affiliated with one of Boston's teaching hospitals, and each under the control of a board elected from and by the patients using a particular center. In 1978, there were approximately 750,000 patient visits to the centers, a figure that translates into at least 125,000 individuals.

The health centers have increasingly moved toward the acquisition of stable, full-time professional staff, toward twenty-four hour coverage, and toward following their patients throughout the health care delivery system — in the health center, the hospital, long-term care facilities, and the home. They all provide a comprehensive array of primary care services appropriate to their size, including obstetrics, gynecology and family planning, pediatrics, and internal medicine.

All centers have appropriate ancillary services on site or by arrangement with outside labs or hospitals. All have social service and dentistry; all but two offer nutrition on site.

How well the centers are working in terms of patient convenience and confidence, professional quality, and resource economy is now the subject of a comprehensive study. The study will pay particular attention to their governance by consumer boards. This trait is attributable to the centers' origin in the poverty program of the late 1960s, all of whose creations were designed as a means of empowering previously inert populations.[4]

The medical profession, which still expects to run services for people who provide illnesses, has looked askance at this aspect of health centers. Writings abound describing the distracting effect of consumer-professional conflict, the demoralization of physicians confronted with complaints about housing conditions rather than bodily disease, and administrators who cannot maintain proper medical or financial records.[5] On the other side, many advocates of neighborhood health centers value them because of their form rather than their performance — because they empower the weak; because they employ the poor; because they give minorities control over institutions.[6] Those advocates resist any inquiry into the centers' contribution to the health of their users.

In my judgment both the critics and the advocates are wrong. The issue is not ideological. As a matter of fact, consumer control — which so far as I know is unique to American primary health centers because of a combination of historical accidents — can be shown to be the most effective way to provide appropriate, inexpensive, and high quality medical care. The current Boston study is testing that hypothesis. It breaks down into three components: first, consumers are more concerned than are professionals with patient convenience; second, consumers can best decide questions for which science has no answers; and third, the very activity of managing one's health care is psychologically and, therefore, physically salubrious.

CONSUMERS ARE CONCERNED WITH PATIENT CONVENIENCE

It is generally believed that the demand for high style treatment of disease comes from consumers who seek the magic bullet — for whom a pound of cure is worth an ounce of prevention. Although it is certainly true that consumer expectations have risen unrealistically, they have done so in response to the promise extended by scientific medicine.[7] Only because the consumer has been led to believe that she or he will receive better care at a downtown hospital do such consumers and their families journey ten miles for attention that could better be obtained at a primary care facility within walking distance of home. In general, the consumer no more wants to be hospitalized for tests than she or he wants to be bled. Both are concoctions of providers.

Of course, people should be able to obtain the most advanced treatment that is appropriate. But most interventions to diagnose or care for prolonged disorders are not urgent; their use can be gradual, exhausting first every technique that can be undertaken in a primary care facility rather than setting off the whole battery of probes and treatments that are available at the highest technological level.

A consumer board has several motivations for a gradual approach to its patients' problems. In the first place, assuming its finances are not distorted by too many nonpaying users of its facilities, it will want to derive income from providing service through its own facilities rather than referring patients elsewhere. This is particularly true if its patients are prepaid members of the center following the pattern set by HMOs, where too many hospital referrals will deplete the organization's resources.

In addition, consumer representatives on boards are aware that the users of the center vastly prefer to have their needs met close to home. Since only facilities of a modest style can be so decentralized, their use is less expensive per patient visit than those of a general hospital, at least in Boston.

Finally, consumers are likely to be willing to exchange the luxury of department store variety for neighborhood accessibility without inordinate delays. Most consumers are aware that they must trade some comprehensiveness for the convenience of having services available locally. While all the neighborhood health centers in the city of Boston offer medical services to children and adults of all ages, they are limited in the specialty services they provide.

Consumer boards that are faced with constituencies of unrequitable needs will almost always elect to meet as many prevalent ones as possible within the limits of their resources. Obviously, kidney dialysis does not commend itself to them as much as pediatrics. And who is better able to decide which services should have priority than people who know how many sick children there are in the neighborhood compared to the number of bad kidneys? Their decisions are also likely to achieve more acceptance by their neighbors than those of a professional who may tell people what is good for them without trying to enlist their understanding or agreement.

The range of services at the centers discloses consumer input in yet another way. They are not simply a local version of what is offered by hospital outpatient departments. They show a tendency toward holistic approaches seldom available at more sophisticated levels. More than half the neighborhood health centers in Boston offer services in family planning, nutrition, dentistry, social service, and mental health. Almost as many provide optometry and ophthalmology. All provide instruction in self-care either through formal programs or as part of regular encounters. The effectiveness of such education in this critical area is still to be assessed. Only a few offer minor surgery, orthopedics, or rheumatology. Of course, such services would be of vast benefit at the local level. But they are frequently foregone simply because they are expensive — a penny wise, pound foolish policy that is costly in money and in spirit.

Consumer boards of the sort I am discussing are seldom faced with the kind of excruciating ethical issue that Sissela Bok describes in Chapter 3 because they are dealing with primary level care. Nevertheless, the problems to which those boards become accustomed — weighing costs and benefits and demands and resources — are not unlike more cosmic dilemmas. Acquainting larger numbers of people with the ingredients of such issues can only help in steering our health system in more sensible directions — allocating resources to more appropriate procedures, relieving disabling discomforts rather than prolonging lives beset with painful, incurable illness or enhancing mobility rather than devoting resources to dubious miracle techniques.

CONSUMERS CAN BEST DECIDE QUESTIONS FOR WHICH SCIENCE HAS NO ANSWERS

Of course, high style providers often assert that money is saved at neighborhood health centers by skimping on the quality of care, as if their clientele could choose among all existing facilities. Jack Geiger calls this criticism "the Marie Antoinette view of health care delivery." The charge would be more telling if we knew that people treated by hospitals or general practitioners receive better care than those who use neighborhood health centers. The depressing truth is that we do not know that a majority of the most common medical interventions are useful;[8] someone has to make a decision based on inadequate evidence. Arguably, consumers are in a better position to do so than providers. They are less caught up than physicians in the notion that mortality can be conquered, or, as someone said, "Death is un-American." They do not share the motivation that science, if not patient care, will be advanced by further treatment. And they are not anxious — at least yet — about malpractice liability for withholding doubtful procedures. To be sure, interventions of demonstrated benefit such as hip replacement and cataract removal should be accessible. But it is equally important to refrain from subjecting patients to distressing treatments that are not known to be efficacious.

Massachusetts last year enacted a patient's bill of rights.[10] It has a provision that requires physicians who diagnose breast cancer to disclose to the victim the several therapies available. The president of the Massachusetts Medical Society commented: "This one provision is difficult. It implies that the patient has the wisdom to make a decision. But the patient hasn't the wisdom to make a decision when it isn't established by scientific evidence . . .."[11]

Who, one wonders, does have that wisdom? In the law, it has long been established that inscrutable decisions should be entrusted to the common sense of ordinary people. "Midway, complicated and doubtful causes . . . go to the jury," Justice Holmes said.[12]

MANAGING ONE'S HEALTH CARE IS SALUBRIOUS

Although there have been studies of neighborhood health centers showing that they are in many places widely accepted by their users and effective and economical in their operation,[13] no study so far as I know has been conducted to ascertain what effect managing one's health care system has on one's health. Yet logic supports the conclusion that active participation therein is itself the healthiest activity one can pursue.

It is a truism that understanding and mastery of one's environment strengthens one's ego. Every educational process in our society is based on the premise that the development of knowledge and skill enlarges life, thus enabling people to develop their potentialities and increase their capacity for joyous living. Just as learning how to use a telephone or bank enables people to overcome feelings of helplessness, understanding the process of a disease and enlisting patients in the fight against it are mighty weapons for cure.[14] In *Anatomy of an Illness*, Norman Cousins recounts how he was beset by a rare degenerative disease. When he was told that the chance of recovery was one in five hundred, Cousins says, "It seemed clear to me that if I was to be that one in five hundred I had better be something more than a passive observer."[15] He then recounts how he substituted vitamins for sedatives, a hotel for the hospital, laughter for dependence — and recovered.

If participating in one's own healing is an effective therapy, so too may participation — even control — of the health system by its users enhance its effectiveness. It becomes their property. No longer — at least at the primary care level — are users confronted with a system that alienates them.

This was the theory behind the policy advanced during the Poverty Program, which recognized that the inability of the poor to use simple cultural artifacts, much less the more elaborate institutions of society, produces feelings of helplessness and anomie. President Johnson said in his State of the Union Address in 1964: "The central problem is to protect and restore man's satisfaction in belonging to a community where he can find security and significance."

Similarly, Robert Kennedy told the Congress later that same year that existing social welfare agencies

> plan programs for the poor, not with them. Part of the sense of helplessness and futility comes from the feeling of powerlessness to affect the operations of these organizations. The community action programs must basically change these organizations by building into the program real representation for the poor. This bill calls for "maximum feasible participation of the residents." This means the involvement of the poor in planning and implementing programs; giving them a real voice in their institutions.[16]

The theory has no less an ancestor than Thomas Jefferson. In his view, public freedom — or "happiness" as he used the word in the Declaration of Independence — was the realization of self through active participation in the basic societal decisions that affect one's life.[17] Interesting too is Jefferson's espousal of "ward" organization. In it he saw the opportunity for people to act directly rather than through representatives to shape their lives. He advised people to use organizations at first only for a single purpose "They will soon show for what others they are the best instruments."[18]

Jefferson's insight is confirmed by consumer control of health centers in Boston. Who knows but what they may prove to be the best instruments for the governance of the entire health care system? But that result will not come about quickly. The establishment has an enduring suspicion of popular government.

No one has ever been thoroughly convinced of the soundness of democracy. In our public affairs we have always lurched between belief in popular government and benevolent despotism.[19] Adlai Stevenson exhorted us to trust the people,[20] and he may have believed it. Jimmy Carter thinks the president should be elected for one six-year term to take politics out of the presidency, and in 1980 he surely believes it.

SUMMARY

It is no surprise, then, that we tend to doubt lay competence when it comes to health. For a hundred years, medicine has been regarded as its principal bulwark, and medicine is incontrovertibly an esoteric subject. Dominant as the previous century is in shaping current thought and conduct, however, we will not forever be under its spell. I am convinced that if our national policy can escape its present domination by high style providers — if it can come to see consumer control as a congenital strength rather than a weakness of the American health care system — then such a mechanism can greatly facilitate progress toward creation of a health care system whose appropriate interventions we can afford.

NOTES

1. *Social Security Bulletin* 41, no. 7 (July 1978).
2. President Carter's proposal for a cap on hospital expenditures, for example, was defeated in Congress in 1979. *The Boston Globe*, November 16, 1979, p. 3.
3. Senator Kennedy's approach to this problem is disappointing. His latest national health insurance proposal would honor all charges by a general hospital but only certain costs in preventive care. Senate Bill 1720, 96th Cong., 1st sess., secs. 201 and 205. See, to the contrary, Karen Davis, "A New Approach to Health Care Delivery," in *Health and the War on Poverty* (Washington, D.C., 1979).
4. Robert Hollister et al., "Neighborhood Health Centers as a Social Movement," in his fine collection, *Neighborhood Health Centers* (Lexington, Mass., 1974), p. 14.
5. Jack Geiger, "Community Control or Community Conflict," in Hollister, *Neighborhood Health Centers*, p. 133.
6. Des Callan et al., "NENA: Community Control in a Bind," in Hollister, *Neighborhood Health Centers*, p. 143; Jack Elinson et al., "A Sociomedical View of Neighborhood Health Centers," in Hollister, *Neighborhood Health Centers*, p. 123; and Public Health Service, USDHEW, *Final Report 1968-1976: Review of Federally Supported Neighborhood Health Centers* (Rockville, Md., 1977).
7. The town of Framingham, Massachusetts, recently voted to appropriate $60,000 to enable one of its firefighters to have a new heart transplanted in the understanding that the procedure was necessary to save his life. After he was examined at the Stanford Medical Center in California, doctors

concluded that the procedure would not benefit him. See *The Boston Globe*, October 11, 1979, p. 1.

8. Ivan Illich, *Medical Nemesis* (New York, 1977).
9. At least in declaring how HMOs should be organized, Congress appears to have harbored such a notion, since it required that at least one-third of the membership of the policymaking body should be members of the HMO and include an "equitable representation" of any medically underserved population served by the HMO. 42 U.S.C. 300e (c) (6) (A).
10. St. 1979, c. 214, now Mass. Gen. Laws c. 111, s. 70E.
11. *The Boston Globe*, August 20, 1979, p. 16.
12. O. W. Holmes, Jr., *The Common Law* (Boston, 1948), 42nd printing, p. 160.
13. E.g., Camille Orso, "Delivering Ambulatory Health Care: The Successful Experience of an Urban Neighborhood Health Center," *Medical Care* 17, no. 2 (February 1979): 111-26.
14. Leonard Small, *The Briefer Psychotherapies*, rev. ed. (New York, 1979), pp. 147-48; Berkman and Syme, "Social Networks, Host Resistance and Mortality," *American Journal of Epidemiology* 109 (1979): 186-204.
15. Norman Cousins, *Anatomy of an Illness* (New York, 1979), quote on p. 31.
16. House Committee on Education and Labor, Hearings on Economic Opportunity Act 1964, pp. 207ff.
17. Hannah Arendt, *On Revolution* (New York, 1963), pp. 234-59.
18. Thomas Jefferson, letters to Samuel Kercheval, July 12 and September 5, 1816; letter to Joseph C. Cahell, February 2, 1816.
19. Daniel P. Moynihan, *Maximum Feasible Misunderstanding* (New York, 1969).
20. Adlai Stevenson, *The New America* (New York, 1957), p. 227.

Chapter 10

Controlling Hospital Costs

Maurice Lazarus

As has been set out in earlier chapters of this book, health care costs are consuming an ever larger share of gross national product in developed countries. Europe is experiencing the same escalation in costs as the United States. This is true in Germany, where national sickness insurance has a long tradition since it was started by Bismarck in 1890. It is true in Sweden, where the government runs the hospitals and employs the physicians. In both these countries health expenditures take a larger share of gross national product than in the United States.

Similar escalations of health care costs are occurring in all the other European countries with the sole exception of Great Britain. There, with stringent central budget control, the cost of the National Health Service has remained a constant percent of the gross national product, substantially below our own. This has been achieved by careful rationing of health care services, queuing for elective surgery, restrictive use of new technology, and stringent control of the number of hospital beds and their usage. The health plan developed from the wartime conditions of scarcity and has survived and is accepted by the British public today. Mortality and morbidity rates in Britain indicate that it has been and continues to be a successful program. No one at the Seminar, however (not even the British), felt that it would be possible for any other country to replicate this experience. The National Health Service came into being in Britain at a particularly auspicious time, and the population has been educated to use the service effectively over a thirty year period.

Political leaders elsewhere are almost unanimous in their condemnation of the cost explosion in health costs and are searching for ways to contain it. Hospital costs are an obvious target for outside efforts to control medical expense. They represent the largest segment of costs — approximately $80 billion of the $200 billion spent on health care. The growth in hospital costs has been 4.5 percent greater than the inflation of medical prices. Hospital usage has not increased as measured in inpatient days in the last several years; rather what is done in our hospitals drives costs up. The number of lab tests has grown at a rate of 15 percent per year and now accounts for approximately $15 billion. Another $8 to $9 billion is spent on diagnostic radiological procedures.

What lies behind this expansion of procedures? In the first place, public expectations of what the medical profession can accomplish are fed by incessant news of new technologies, new procedures, new miracle drugs, often engendering unrealistic demands from physicians. It is difficult for physicians to resist patients' pressure and particularly difficult in the litigious atmosphere in which they practice. But it is the physician alone who is equipped to put into perspective for the patient what is realistically possible and to do it in a way that does not call forth unnecessary diagnostic testing and unproven, undocumented procedures. If physicians are paid on a fee for service basis (the predominant custom in the United States), they have very little incentive to impose these restraints. Quite the contrary, they have good reason to explore at whatever cost the patient's unrealistic expectations.

Second, hospitals are under similar pressures, but in addition, most have a long tradition of doing everything that can be done to save the life of the person who enters its doors. As new technology develops (and it has been exploding) and as it becomes more and more difficult to define the fine line between life and death, more and more procedures are prescribed.

The pressures to spend far outpace the pressures to control cost. Trying to control costs from outside the system invariably leads to dislocation of services and supply. We are left with the challenge how to try to control costs within the system. How can we manage the public's expectations?

At Salzburg there seemed to be a unanimous feeling that changing the delivery systems would not control costs; cost control can more effectively be accomplished within the existing delivery system. We delude ourselves if we think that national health insurance, for example, is a panacea for controlling escalating costs. Unfortunately, there is no quick macro-fix. But there are some lessons to be learned from experience, particularly from the prepaid group practices that have developed in the last forty years.

The health maintenance organizations, such as the Kaiser-Permanente system, are good examples. These are organized systems of health care. They provide comprehensive service through a group of physicians within a defined geographic area on a fixed fee prepayment basis. These organizations have been able to reduce costs by appropriate use of health professionals for outpatient service. But more importantly, they have substantially reduced the rate of hospitalization. Their premium levels range from 10 to 40 percent below community-rated insurance plans that are delivering health care in the traditional fee for service manner. The physicians in these groups have an incentive to keep their patients' expectations down to realistic levels. They are usually employed on a salary and bonus arrangement. The bonus depends upon the success of the plan in keeping its costs below premium income. What the plan must pay for hospitalization of its members is an important part of its cost. Therefore, the physicians exhaust most possibilities of outpatient treatment before sending a member to a hospital. This, of course, is not true in emergency situations.

Health maintenance organizations now have approximately 8 million members. They have been expanding rapidly, as have other forms of prepaid group practices. The success of the expansion depends not only on their cost effectiveness but also on their ability to maintain a quality of care satisfactory to their members.

It is true that health maintenance organizations do not service a cross-section of the population. Their members are mostly employed people and their families. Few patients are over sixty-five years old. But even if the statistics are corrected for these demographic differences, health maintenance organizations are still more cost effective. Their savings have occurred primarily because physicians have the responsibility for the cost of the system, and they are rewarded for keeping those costs under control.

I think a similar set of incentives can work effectively in controlling hospital costs. The first step in the process is to put the physicians in charge of hospital costs in addition to being responsible for patient care, research, and teaching. Of course, that cannot be done effectively without decentralizing responsibility. The Johns Hopkins Medical Center has completed that transformation. Each chief of clinical service now has the responsibility for costs. He or she is charged for the hospital services the patients use, for the costs of the nursing care they receive, and for the space the chief and his or her staff occupy.

The organizational model is not new to industry. Most complex institutions organize themselves into profit centers, each standing on its own as if it were a separate little business. But in a hospital setting, this is not so simple. If physicians are to be responsible for the costs of their service, they must know what those costs are, and they must understand and believe that they are accurate and reasonably assessed.

The acquisition of this knowledge will entail a complete renovation of current hospital accounting systems. Present so-called functional accounting is an outgrowth of the hospitals' ancient tradition of charging the full costs of the hospital's operation to those patients who could afford to pay. These costs were originally assessed in the form of a day rate. Then as day rates advanced, more and more ancillary services were billed directly. This procedure in no way reflects actual costs.

The day rate now represents about 50 percent of hospital charges. It is the residue of total costs that is left after the ancillary charges have been recovered. Further, the day rate charge is the same for each day a person stays in the hospital. Actually, the first day's stay, which includes the cost of admitting and discharging a patient, is normally the most expensive day. The second and third days are probably more expensive than the ninth and tenth days, because more intensive nursing care is required early in a hospital visit.

The Massachusetts Eye and Ear Infirmary made a careful analysis of its daily costs. It has set separate rates for each day of stay that more closely resemble the costs. But on the whole, hospital accounting today does not effectively surface the cost of individual services that are rendered. Even the ancillary charges usually do not reflect accurate cost information. This means that if an organizational form is to be set up where the physicians are responsible for the cost of their operations, a separate set of accounting procedures must be developed that will reasonably and accurately reflect the cost of each service.

If physicians are to be held responsible for the cost of their operations, the chief of each service will require administrative support to be able to handle the additional work effectively. A new echelon of management will need to be trained to handle the administrative supervision of the department and to become familiar with the new accounting procedures.

The charging mechanism to patients must also be changed to a fee schedule predetermined each year for each diagnosis rather than the present day rate plus ancillary care. The present rate for diagnosis would include all services that the hospital renders for that particular malady. Such a plan is now being initiated in New Jersey. For it to be effective, a detailed diagnosis must be made of each patient entering the hospital. A patient coming in for an appendectomy who has a history of heart disease and diabetes would be charged a different rate than a person coming in for the same operation with no prior history of potential complications. Most teaching hospitals have detailed diagnostic records of their patients. It should be possible to develop equitable charges that matched diagnoses. The charge that a patient paid would be the same whether he or she stayed in the hospital three days or eight days and regardless of the ancillary services received. Inasmuch as the physician determines the treatment and dictates the length of stay, he or she would be in charge of the patient's treatment in just the same way as today.

Finally, there would be an incentive for physicians to manage the costs. That incentive would be a share in the saving between the preset patient charge and the cost of treating that patient. Each chief of service would be in charge of what is known in industry as a profit center. Each service chief and the full- and part-time physicians who work with her or him must have a stake in seeing that they manage a patient's care as economically as possible. They as a group would derive the benefits for so doing and as individuals would be paid a portion of the profits. They would thus have the same incentives as physicians in a health maintenance organization for keeping the costs within bounds.

Such a program must include one safeguard — the careful policing of the quality of care patients receive in hospital. The need exists to be constantly alert that improper shortcuts are avoided and that proper protocols are followed. The review function of PSROs would be even more important than it is today.

In order to place physicians in charge of controlling costs and to give them incentives for doing so, we must reorganize our hospitals. The organizational structure must be changed so that the physician has the necessary administrative assistance to be able to discharge his total responsibility. The accounting systems must be changed so that we have reasonably accurate costs for each service that is performed in hospital. The billing structure must be changed from a charge for service to a charge for the total treatment of a particular diagnosis. The incentive systems in hospitals must be changed so that physicians share in the savings they are able to effect through a careful monitoring of the patients' length of stay and the use of ancillary services.

Under such a system we should get much more efficient use of facilities. As hospitals are run more efficiently, the threat of increased outside regulation will be reduced, and hospitals will retain freedom to decide their own futures.

It would be a mistake to underestimate the complexity of making these changes. At the present time, hospitals are burdened with special accounting requirements to meet Medicaid, Blue Cross, and other insurance procedures. The present complications of complying with regulatory directives are enormous. Initially, a parallel system of accounts would have to be developed. Profit centers would be created with cost allocations that minimize overhead assessments. A new echelon of management must participate in this development. They must understand how these costs are distributed and how they can be controlled. New supervisory relationships may have to be developed for nursing staffs and operating rooms.

These changes are complex. But I believe such a drastic overhaul is called for if we are going to check this most volatile element in rising health costs.

Chapter 11

Account of Proceedings at the Salzburg Seminar

Mitchell Goldman, Christopher Robbins, and Other Fellows

The 190th session of the Salzburg Seminar comprised thirty-eight fellows and seven faculty from seventeen countries and a wide spread of disciplines and responsibilities. Formal presentations on the general background and on particular country organizations with opportunities for questions and discussion were given by faculty members and some fellows. Seminars on a wide variety of aspects of health care organization, as well as more informal group discussion, occurred throughout the period. The second week was substantially taken up by syndicate discussions organized by the fellows to examine particular aspects of the problem. The syndicate reports were made to the whole group and were discussed there, but they should not be read as agreed conclusions of the full Seminar.

THE ROLE OF HEALTH SERVICES IN A MODERN SOCIETY

Health and well-being cannot be regarded as merely the outcome of health services, nor do further inputs in service always produce measurable gains in either. Society faced by the continuing escalation of costs must be concerned to restrain any part that appears unproductive whether new or long continuing. Any such restraint must involve the political system, and different systems will handle it in different ways. Questions of individual freedom inevitably arise when the system seeks to reach equity within overall limitations on the total of service available. Different societies respond in ways that reflect the history of development of their political organization both central and local. Custom may permit controls that are acceptable in the USSR, Scandinavia, or Britain that would be rejected in France, North America, or Australia. Other countries, such as Tanzania or China with more recent development and different cultures, may be far more rigorous in their controls on the use of exiguous resources.

The development of a sanitary environment, adequate nutrition, and appropriate housing together with employment and education both in both general and health matters have been mainly responsible for health improvement in industrialized societies. Their influence is not entirely spent, since atmospheric pollution and newer problems of chemicals in the environment and exposure to ionizing radiations require new safeguards. In developing countries most of these gains have yet to be made, and as they are made, they will impart new problems in population dynamics. This aspect of health promotion is expensive and often attainable only in the long term, but it does not depend on voluntary individual response so much as on regulatory controls that governments can devise.

The recent recognition of the overriding importance of human lifestyle in health promotion stems largely from the Canadian report associated with the name of Marc Lalonde, former minister of health. Many studies have shown how much the choice of foods, avoidance of smoking, abuse of alcohol, overweight, restraint in driving, and physical activity promote better health during a longer life. Recent studies in the United States and Finland, reported by David Hamburg, include experimental evidence of the lower atherogenic effect of the modified diet now followed there.

The desired changes in lifestyle are not such as can be secured by regulatory means, but educational programs and the provision of greater opportunities for healthful activities such as regular exercise require government support. Much of the promotion required is nonmedical, involving, for example, educational and social services. A tendency to "medicalization" of deviance from optimal lifestyles may be actually harmful if it reduces input from other sources such as social services. Nevertheless, constraints on promotion of health-damaging factors in society such as excessive consumption of alcohol, the use of tobacco products, or ill-advised choice of foods, as described in the McGovern Report, are inescapable, if unpopular, responsibilities of governments. Government action to replace tobacco culture and processing is essential. Certain individual restraints such as speed limits, the wearing of crash helmets by motorcyclists and of seatbelts by motorists, and the avoidance of alcohol intake by drivers require courageous government intervention, which some countries have already undertaken.

Questions of availability and justification for application of new technology were examined by syndicates on Policy Formulation and Health Planning. General questions about new technology were raised at Salzburg on the scientific side by David Hamburg and on the ethical side by Sissela Bok. They discussed the special problem of controlling the use of costly technologies for palliation or doubtful amelioration of incurable conditions. Means for assessing such questions are needed, and they may not be left to individual professional judgment, accepted as that practice is. Not only must the professional base used to define policies be broadened, but nonhealth professionals and consumers must be introduced into such decision-making.

All countries are moving toward a regional planning system that both permits rational and economic development of district services and deters wasteful duplication of expensive facilities whether of beds or new technological services — for example, review of proposals for new facilities by Health Systems Agencies in the United States, provinces in Canada, *departements* in France, and *Länder* in Germany. Fully planned and administered services such as those in the United Kingdom, New Zealand, and the Soviet Union control development and staffing within regional or national plans.

The regionalization process is usually linked to a planning process, the purpose of which is to provide a mechanism to make the difficult decisions of resource allocation. The Syndicate on Planning examined the planning process and generally concluded that setting priorities in the health care sector must not be limited to capital expenditures. Consideration must be given to psychosocial and economic factors as well. The relationship between health expenditures and the rest of the economy must be evaluated if sensible decisions are to be made.

The Syndicate on Planning described a more general methodology comprising the multidimensional aspects of the planning process. Needs must be identified in order to define goals in any society. But data is generally insufficient to support reliable judgments. Consideration must be given to the political and social attitudes that dominate the selection of objectives and strategies in any country. Finally, evaluation must be a part of any process to insure that the system continues to improve and to identify better ways of delivering service and allocating resources.

SPECIAL PROBLEMS: PRIMARY CARE AND CARE OF THE ELDERLY

The fellows felt that two areas merited special attention because of their implications for resource allocation in developing and developed countries. While each topic is exceptionally broad, a few specific problems in each area were addressed.

Primary Care

Countries were seen to vary widely in their systems for development of primary care. Examples were given of the extension of the work of specialists outside hospitals into community care, such as the primary care role of many internists, pediatricians, and gynecologists in North America; the use of specialist community clinics staffed by physicians not attached to hospitals in Israel; the polyclinics of the Soviet Union or health centers of Yugoslavia; the "office" consultations with specialists in West Germany; and the children's clinics conducted by community pediatricians in many countries. The reverse situation can be seen in the direct access of patients for first contact in hospital outpatient facilities in Sweden. Some countries employ a referral system from primary to secondary care (United Kingdom, Denmark, New Zealand) and others apply financial sanctions through larger copayments from patients who seek service from specialists direct (Australia).

The Syndicate on Primary Care emphasized not only the value of strengthening primary care resources but also the importance of communication between professionals engaged therein and their colleagues in hospitals. Haim Doron had made a special point of this development in Israel, where, as in the USSR or Poland, some authority over primary care physicians is given to hospital chiefs of service. The British emphasize a continuing educational process between hospital- and community-based health professionals in a district. Britain also uses a more organized multiprofessional team, based where possible on health centers as described by Marsh and Kaim Candle. Admittedly, the ideal relationship is not always present, and the absence of authority may permit some very poor quality service to continue.

The Syndicate on Primary Care also addressed the problems in terms of two specific themes related to the allocation of resources. First, the development of adequate primary care services is essential for efficient resource allocation. Second, prevention and early intervention reduce the abuse of inpatient hospital services. The delivery of primary care services was examined from two perspectives — the collaboration between primary care physicians and specialists in a local clinic and the team approach to the delivery of primary care services.

The general practitioner-specialist relationship needs to be improved by upgrading the status of the "generalist" relative to the specialist in the eyes of the medical profession and the public. This can be done in several ways. First, education at the undergraduate and postgraduate levels should enhance the role of the general practitioner. Continuing education programs for the general practitioner must be developed. Second, through the development of research programs and professional organizations, general practice can gain the status of a specialty. Finally, general practitioners' compensation should approximate most specialists'.

The team approach to primary care services was considered an important aspect of effective delivery of service. A team is necessary to carry out the broad mandates of a primary care service — prevention, diagnosis, treatment, and rehabilitation. The primary care team should include a variety of providers, such as midwives, public health nurses, health visitors, and social workers. Through a team approach, the patient can better be seen as a whole individual. In addition, consideration can be given to the patient's social, environmental, and emotional conditions. The structure, organization, and financing of the primary care services must support the growth of primary care and provide incentives for practitioners to work in teams, not in isolation. The upgrading of the status of general practitioners and the development of primary care teams will strengthen primary care service delivery.

Care of the Elderly

The number of older people is increasing in the developed countries. Projections of 10 to 20 percent of the populations by the end of a decade are not uncommon. As this population increases, the demands on the health care system will increase, since the aged tend to use a disproportionate amount of health care services relative to their numbers in the population. For example, the United States spends three times more per capita on persons over sixty-five than on those under sixty-five, and the United Kingdom spends four and a half times as much on those over sixty-five as on those between fifteen and sixty-four. With these resource demands, there is a need to identify how services can be provided to this group without unfairly diminishing resources available to others.

The Syndicate on Care of the Elderly concluded that more varied resources were needed than those of the health profession. Many social components in support for the elderly also contribute to their health maintenance, including financial support, special housing, and help in the home, often with provision of meals. Countries use institutional provision in very different ways — some, like Sweden, have large hostel and hospital provision; some, like Denmark, give special statutory rights to more homelike provision in nursing homes; some, like Germany, place special emphasis on appropriate housing; and some, like Britain, make their chief effort in support in the home.

The development of a medical specialty of geriatrics is best seen in Britain, but Denmark also has a "long-term care" specialty. Much depends on physicians' recognition of the predominantly social needs of the elderly sick. The balance between social welfare, housing, and health care expenditures was particularly considered.

The underlying premises of planning services for the elderly are threefold: (1) all persons should be helped to remain independent and to assume maximum responsibility for their own well-being; (2) services provided for the elderly should enable them to remain at home for as long as possible; (3) health care system and social programs must be jointly responsible for providing care for the elderly. Present services inadequately address (1) the psychological aspects of aging manifested in drug misuse, alcoholism, and suicide; (2) the need for social service and environmental support; (3) the need for community services instead of institutional services; and (4) the problems of isolation, loneliness, and depression of the single elderly.

The needs of the elderly could be effectively met by a consideration of housing needs, appropriate institutional placement, and home care services. An array of housing alternatives that are especially adapted for the elderly and their differing levels of functional disability are necessary. Resource allocation policies should recognize that with such an array of housing, fewer long stay facilities would be required. Social welfare and health services information and coordination should be handled by either a public health nurse or a social worker. Finally, services for the elderly must have a full complement of in home services including home nursing, personal care, meals on wheels, house cleaning, food shopping, home repair, chiropody, and services that foster companionship.

Primary care services are essential for the elderly to avoid over-utilization of hospital services. Early intervention will be an effective means of containing costs by treating medical problems before they become serious. In addition, problems of vision and hearing care must be identified early to insure that the elderly can function at maximum levels. The primary care team should also be aware of the need for the special consultant services of a geriatrician whose services are integrated into the acute care hospital.

MEASURES AFFECTING THE FUTURE OF HEALTH CARE

Prevention

In industrialized societies, new developments offer more in human terms from longer life in better health than in economic terms from saving life. There is much to be done by preventing accidents, which exact an especially heavy toll on the young — perhaps 10 to 20 percent of years of life lost before normal retiring age. Much could be done to prevent other premature deaths from ischaemic heart disease or from cancer (diet, exercise, smoking), but these and other longer-term benefits will not be reflected in short-term reductions in health care expenditures. The clientele requiring these short-term expenditures are already here and damaged. Human rather than cost benefits may be the main outcome.

The Syndicate on Disease Prevention examined the various aspects of a health policy seeking the prevention of illness in developed countries where infectious disease has been reduced and the dominant problems are those related to lifestyle (e.g., smoking, alcoholism, drug abuse and misuse). Emphasis on environmental control is emerging as a major and costly method of prevention. Human genetics, on the other hand, offers new opportunities for prevention, especially in the early stages of life. From the examination of preventive approaches to health, the syndicate concluded that (1) national illness prevention efforts must be interdepartmental; (2) priorities should be set by effectiveness of treatment as well as seriousness and magnitude of the problem; (3) ethical dimensions must be included in an analysis of actions; and (4) disease prevention strategies may not reduce costs but could reduce premature death.

Education of Health Professionals and the Public

The Syndicate on Education considered the needs of both the health professions and the public. Greater emphasis on the whole human problem in ill health is needed, and its submersion by high technology must be prevented. More use of joint educational programs between the various professions is desirable. Education in health should be part of the general educational curriculum, and special resources such as the Open University in Britain should be used.

Specialization may be necessary as part of the progress in biomedical science, but it should not be allowed to prevent suitable exchanges and satisfactory career development in the sciences and technologies complementary to medicine. The Netherlands is currently reviewing this issue.

There is an uneasy air of tension between the family of professions in many countries, partly due to the autocratic tendencies of physicians and the growing assertiveness of other professionals. The physician's assumption of a right to leadership in all circumstances is no longer accepted, especially by nurses and social workers. The syndicate felt strongly that the current political and planning processes were inadequate to identify the key issues and to provide the necessary leadership to effect significant changes in the manpower education policies of governments. Insufficient awareness of health and illness was considered to be the major obstacle to effective consumer education. The syndicate recommended that (1) professional educators emphasize primary care services, (2) health education for the consumer be integrated into general education, and (3) the public be made aware of cost advantages of self-care.

Research

More vigorous and effective health services research is essential to rational development. Controlled clinical trials offer one method of assessing new methods of diagnosis or treatment, but they are not always applicable and present ethical problems. Nevertheless, there are many examples of widely used methods that have not been validated for selective use or indeed for use at all. Tonsillectomy and surgery for breast cancer or for coronary artery disease are examples. Some obvious advances, such as the use of l-dopa in Parkinsonism, cannot be held back, but even they may be the less well used for lack of a cautious, controlled beginning.

Diagnostic procedures involving expensive new technology may be widely disseminated at great cost before their value and limitations have been properly assessed. The largest recent example is computerized axial tomography, which is an invaluable tool in neurology but is probably used far more widely than is strictly necessary. There have been many other investigations of undoubted benefit in particular situations but of uncertain or even negative value in mass use, such as tonometry for population screening for glaucoma and routine amniocentesis for prenatal diagnosis of Down's syndrome.

In a number of lectures and seminars at Salzburg, David Hamburg traced the exciting history of recent scientific discoveries, particularly in the area of genetics. He forecast astonishing new applications of knowledge that will put tremendous strains on inadequate mechanisms for safe, equitable, and efficient diffusion. America, he said, has developed a terrible health system for the rich that everyone now wants. It was pointed out that it is almost impossible to prevent the application of any new technique once its use becomes possible regardless of its safety or lasting efficacy. Mechanisms for effective monitoring evaluation and research into health systems must be expanded and strengthened if the wild beast of technology is to be tamed. There should be more international sharing in the formulation of science policy.

THE PROBLEM OF THE SCARCITY OF RESOURCES: THE EVOLUTION TOWARD RATIONING HEALTH CARE

It is clear that open-ended funding of health services has already been restricted in various ways in most countries either by queuing, selective development or allocation, or pricing. Some implicit or explicit process of resource allocation has become necessary to all, even though modest growth of health care expenditure may be allowed by some countries. Such limitations have to be made acceptable to all involved — health care consumers and providers alike — and as explicit as possible.

Robert Maxwell set himself the task of explaining how and why the problem of health care expenditure has arisen and what its theoretical and practical implications are. The background to the problem has four main features:

1. Costs have escalated faster than the increase in prosperity in all developed countries. There seems to be a relationship between GNP per capita and the amount spent on health per capita that holds through time. Indeed, GNP per capita is a good predic-

tor of the level of health spending. (No doubt part of the explanation of this trend is that rises in GNP per capita entail increases in discretionary income and in people's inclination to spend more on health care.)

2. There has been a progressive trend from private to public payment for services (including government funding of welfare and other health measures). It may be felt that this process helps to mask the true cost of health care from consumers and providers.
3. Concurrently, there has been a gradual transition from private forms of health care administration to public institutions carrying out these functions.
4. There is no uniform proportion of health care expenditure devoted to hospital services between countries. On the other hand, the split between capital and recurrent expenditure and the proportion devoted to health care personnel remain roughly constant from country to country.

The causes of the rapid rise of health care expenditure can be described as follows:

1. The pattern of disease has changed: health care has more and more often to devote resources to chronic diseases in an aging population that do not cause quick death now that most short-term fatal infectious diseases have been conquered.
2. Small improvements in health now cost more and more, since there are no major inexpensive "conquests" left to make. Both patients and doctors still feel, however, that this expenditure is worthwhile.
3. Advances in technology often lead to increased expenditure by replacing cheaper treatments with more expensive new ones.
4. Both medical professionals and patients have rising expectations about the effectiveness and quality of medical care.
5. After a long period when health work was considered quasi-charitable and low status, the pay of health personnel has caught up. While technological development has generally raised wages elsewhere, the health care system has not benefited from the labor saving that technology has made possible in most industries. Medical care remains a labor-intensive activity like theater or law.
6. Medical professionals have become more specialized and thus more demanding of resources and more highly paid.
7. The transfer of payments from private to public sources has undoubtedly led to more recourse to services.

Governments have responded to these developments by attempting to limit expenditures. (In Canada the proportion of the GNP taken up by health care stood at 7.1 percent in 1976 as it had done in 1970.) The theoretical framework for restrictive government action can be described as follows:

1. Ways of restraining expenditure do exist that operate independently of (and in spite of) whatever remains of the "free" market in health care.
2. Most governments now recognize that rationing is inevitable, cannot be left to the market (for health care supply and demand are not independent), and must flow from supply rather than demand side initiatives.
3. A consensus has emerged in almost all countries in favor of equity. Rationing must not involve unfair financial or geographical barriers to services.

The practical implications are (1) cost control by transferring hospitals to the public sector, by global budgeting, and by price control; and (2) rational management of resources, looking at each sector in turn, to set the total of expenditure deemed acceptable and to work out how effective services are to be channeled to deal with unmet needs. In this sense, the decision to contain costs is "only the beginning of the story."

The Syndicate on Rationing Health Care took its lead from Mr. Maxwell's exposition. The group agreed that rationing has become unavoidable for most developed countries (although some southern European countries still hope to expand and improve services before imposing overall constraints). Nonetheless, the introduction of health care rationing has its paradoxical aspects: First, it involves global or general measures to constrain supply applied to an essentially individualized service based on the patient-doctor relationship. Second, rationing must be introduced before the medical services have even a reasonably complete understanding of unmet health needs and the effective types of care.

The taxonomy of health care adopted by the group included three main categories of intervention by governments to affect health care consumption — market or economic incentives, moral suasion, and bureaucratic planning and budgeting. All these modes of rationing raise problems, but only the last can promise to hit a given expenditure target for two reasons:

First, market interventions aimed at rationing lead either to inequity (cost sharing imposed on consumers), to transfer of demand rather than supply controls (capitation instead of fee for service payments for doctors), or to control of some cost elements but not the volume of consumption itself (price and fee controls). In general, market interventions leave open the possibility that the market will react to them by finding another way of spending the money that the government hopes to save. This is an inherent risk in leaving a degree of economic independence to entrepreneurs, institutions, and suppliers.

Second, moral suasion, while desirable in itself, cannot be used to aim at given expenditure targets. It is persuasive, not mandatory, and it frequently aims at very long-term benefits (e.g., the campaign against smoking) and can only with difficulty compete against pressures on consumers to indulge in immediately gratifying but unhealthy pursuits.

Governments will be led more or less reluctantly to seek consensus for such measures. Global budgeting can be applied rather crudely by setting a fixed prospective budget for all or most health care, based on previous years' expenditure with perhaps an allowance for growth. At the same time it must seek equity between regions and districts on the demographic characteristics of each area, on any available morbidity data, and on utilization of service rates. This more ambitious analytical approach presupposes a regional-district structure that some countries may lack, and it requires for its equitable and efficient operation a system for the transmission of data to the planning authorities from lower administrative tiers and control of planning decisions. At the same time, decisions as to the allocation of available funds among local needs must be entrusted to communities and consumer representatives, for they must live with the chosen range and quality of services.

Global budgeting gives a government the certainty that a total limit will not be exceeded and makes explicit the constraints under which health care will be provided. Combined with more piecemeal measures to control manpower, fees, and prices and to supervise insurance organizations, its effectiveness is undoubted. However, it raises the problems of equity at the point at which services are provided: medical practitioners are not necessarily well equipped to make difficult cost or ethical decisions; or to decide whether to use waiting lists, corporate decision procedures, random allocations, or other devices to fulfill the requirements passed down to them from above. Further, the very process of budgeting tends to freeze a given "mix" of services, ignoring the possibility of service substitution to save money and perhaps generally slowing down the process of service improvement.

A "parallel market" may spring up alongside the public sector to answer the demands of those prepared to pay to circumvent rationing. In most countries, people have the right to use discretionary income to buy these extra services, but a government must not allow a "parallel market" to attract personnel and supplies that it needs for its own public service. However, the very high cost of medical care should deter the majority of people from leaving the public sector frequently for private treatment, particularly if they have traditionally been protected by a satisfactory social-security-based or public health service (as the majority of Europeans have been).

Consideration of global budgeting invites reflection about four questions:

1. How do we aim for a given level of health care expenditure, rather than waiting for stability to be achieved by the "market"?
2. What criteria should be used to ration equitably between regions and districts, and how should regional interests be balanced with central policies?
3. How can various levels of the health care system participate in the formulations of a rationing policy?
4. How do we clarify the ethical problems facing service providers working within a fixed budget and maintain attention to them?

While the general policy of rationing gets under way in the next few years in many developed countries, attempts to contain and control costs through resource management must continue. The Syndicate on Resource Management examined this problem, finding that any strategy would require a good data base, consisting of a simple comprehensive information system rather than a multiplicity.

The cost problem can be split into five areas — hospitals, professional users, capital buildings, manpower, and cost sharing.

1. Hospitals form the most expensive component of most health care systems. Hence we must make better use of hospitals and promote day care surgery, programmed admissions and discharges, and shorter lengths of stay. These measures save costs in hospitals though they may add costs elsewhere in the care system — for instance, in home nursing and other domiciliary services.
2. Doctors have complete clinical autonomy in any health care system and thus directly control much expenditure in hospitals. They must be made aware of the financial outcome of their actions and encouraged in cost-saving methods. This has already been tried for limited services, and experiments are now under-

way to inform clinicians about the cost of the whole service that they prescribe, so that they can make adjustments accordingly.

3. Hospitals have a life of fifty to a hundred years, during which time medical practice may alter radically. Thus, new buildings must be flexible in design.
4. Manpower — particularly medical manpower — is a crucial cost element. With freedom of movement of professionals between countries and overproduction of doctors in some countries, there is clearly room for some form of international planning and control.
5. Cost sharing — from the individual's viewpoint — should be examined for its effect on consumption of services and on service substitution.

The methods discussed depend on good management, which may not be easy to obtain in a nonprofit industry. And the instincts of good management have to compete with self-interest, traditional procedures, genuine belief that thrift diminishes quality, and institutional habits as old as the health care system itself.

CONCLUSION: ETHICAL AND POLITICAL CONSIDERATIONS

A general review of the topics discussed and the conclusions reached must include the ethical and political dimensions of the problems, and these too were examined in some detail. Sissela Bok described the application of ethical understanding to medical problems, emphasizing that ethical dilemmas arise because resources are scarce and information is often very difficult to collect, while human sympathies in turn are often biased or limited.

Rationing in particular involves decisions turning on the contested notions of utility (avoidance or prevention of harm, production or maintenance of benefit) and justice (defense of liberty, fairness, equality). Veracity is also crucial — as the basis of confidence in the administration of rationing itself. Notions of fairness essential to rationing cannot invariably be applied to choices. Recourse to the principle of utility, for example, restricts the individual's right to treatment and care, whatever the long-term prospects for his and other cases. The principle of utility looks for the result of an action in terms of aggregate benefit and may thus conflict with the interests of minorities or of those who have not long to live or who have little or no prospect of a full and fruitful life. As for liberty, medical professions have insisted on their right to choose whom to treat and how. This right can easily conflict with other principles of justice, such as equality of access, adopted by health systems. Under rationing, collectively established policies may sometimes encroach upon freedom so valued by clinicians.

These problems are well illustrated by the question of allocating scarce resources — in renal dialysis and transplantation, for example. The most detailed criteria for the selection of patients for treatment was used in Seattle for renal dialysis and included (1) medical chances of success; (2) geographical location of the subject; (3) his or her financial resources; (4) his or her proven willingness to cooperate; (5) rehabilitation potential; (6) psychological status; and (7) value to the community.

The last criterion raises the problems of viewing a breadwinner as a means to support his or her family, rather than as just an autonomous individual, and viewing people who do not "qualify" for treatment because of their low "social value" as sacrifices to society in the interest of worthier patients. Criterion 6 seems rather hard on the depressed or subnormal, while criteria 3, 4, and 5 similarly pick on characteristics beyond the patient's control. The medical criterion 1 is an effectiveness rule that makes sense in any treatment decision, while criterion 2 simply delimits the responsibility of the unit. But they are the only two criteria that do not raise serious ethical questions.

Instead of using criteria 3 through 7, the service provider may thus prefer to use a waiting list or random allocation system. If there is a drive to provide services for problems like renal failure to all claimants, the U.S. experience shows how very costly this can be and underlines the consideration that vast expenditure on one item will in the future mean starving others.

These considerations demonstrate that where resources are limited, a utility principle that maximizes benefit for most people conflicts with individual rights, the requirements of fairness, and the necessity of autonomy. There is, however, no obvious balance between utility and justice, and there will be many dilemmas that are not readily solved. When rationing is imposed, so too is the obligation to look for less expensive substitutable treatments and in general to direct research toward finding effective answers to prevalent health problems.

The session also included discussion of the political dimensions of the problem of allocating scarce health care resources. To some extent political issues are coterminous with ethical issues — as, for instance, when a government espouses the principle of equity applied to health care. In general, however, political decisions have to take considerable account of the context as well as the consequences of decisions. It is helpful to look at the history of the development of governmental intervention in what was initially a matter between the individual patient and his or her doctor. From modest welfare interventions and private or mutual insurance arrangements, government intervention has grown to include the direct provision of a universal health service, or the management of a sickness insurance scheme covering almost the whole population, or a combination of these, or a multiplicity of ambitious and costly piecemeal interventions in a "free" market. These modes of intervention evolved from certain circumstances: the inadequacy of sickness insurance in the United Kingdom led to public pressure for a National Health Service, whereas in other countries, such as Sweden and New Zealand, universal health services grew up out of a combination of local collective initiatives and a central social policy, the latter utilizing the former to create a widespread and powerful system.

What are the political issues raised, against this background, by the scarcity of health care resources? There can be no single institutional reform applicable to all developed countries. Nonetheless, Italy has chosen to replace its insurance system by a national health service, while France and the Federal Republic of Germany look with interest at some of the centralized budgeting and control techniques in use in a national health service. These principles of management and allocation are most likely to be grafted on to existing structures, which may ultimately be utterly transformed by the process. It is harder to predict the outcome in countries relying heavily on private health insurance: Will they too be persuaded to adopt a form of centralized management of the health care system or continue to rely on piecemeal measures whose overall effect must be fairly unpredictable and highly expensive?

The centralization of the health care system's management flows from the evolution of most governments' responsibility for the service (which now accounts for one-tenth of national expenditure in many countries). However, the political imperatives also indicate a very important role for local communities, which while they cannot settle overall budgets, can take realistic decisions about, for example, the best combination of local resources, the location of facilities, the replacement of out-dated facilities, and the use of "new money." Local decisionmaking could well be reinforced in the United Kingdom, while in the United States it often represents an effective means for the explicit search for consensus and for communal equity. There are two elements in health care management whose importance cannot be overlooked — the consumer (whose voice must find expression at local level) and the elected representative (whose accountability is the key feature of any successful system of resource allocation).

Ethical and political considerations thus point the way toward the implementation of general and particular resource allocation measures. They generally suggest that two major principles be taken into account:

1. In the process of the allocation of scarce resources, we are obliged to consider each individual's needs and not just the aggregate benefit to society of a particular measure. A primary care service, therefore, to which all have access, is an indispensable part of a health care system, however constrained its resources.
2. Once the global and regional allocations have been carried out, planning of many basic facilities must be decided at the local level, so that consumers can determine the nature of the service that so closely affects their lives.

About the Editor and Contributors

Herbert P. Gleason, secretary of the Salzburg Seminar, practices law in Boston, Massachusetts. Previously, he was Corporation Counsel for Boston and Chairman of its Board of Health and Hospitals.

Sissela Bok is Lecturer on Medical Ethics at the Harvard Medical School. She holds a doctorate in philosophy from Harvard University. A member of the Board of Directors of the Hastings Institute of Society, Ethics and the Life Science, she is the author of *Lying: Moral Choice in Private and Public Life* and of "Freedom and Risk," which appeared in *Daedalus.*

Haim R. Doron, M.D., M.P.H., is Chairman of the Health Insurance Institution of the General Federation of Labour in Israel, and Head of the Community Medicine Department in the Tel Aviv University Medical School. He also serves as Professor of Community Medicine at the university.

Mitchell Goldman is Managing Director of G.L.S. Associates, Inc., health care consultants in Philadelphia.

Sir George Godber, D.M., K.C.B., served for thirty-four years in the

British Ministry of Health and was Chief Medical Officer of the ministry from 1960 to 1973. In addition, he was a member of the Executive Board of the World Health Organization for ten years. Most recently, he was Chairman of the Health Education Council (1977–1978) and a member of the Management Committee of the King Edward's Hospital Fund for London (1973–1977).

David A. Hamburg, M.D., is a Professor of Health Policy and Management in the Kennedy School of Government, Harvard University. From 1975 to 1980, he was President of the Institute of Medicine, National Academy of Sciences. Dr. Hamburg is former head of the Department of Psychiatry at Stanford University Medical School.

Maurice Lazarus is Chairman of the Finance Committee of Federated Department Stores. He serves on the boards of many business and charitable corporations, including the Harvard Community Health Plan, the Massachusetts General Hospital, the Overseers of Harvard College, and the Harvard/M.I.T. Division of Health Sciences and Technology.

Robert J. Maxwell is Secretary of the King Edward's Hospital Fund for London. Previously, he was Administrator to the Special Trustees, St. Thomas' Hospital in London, and consultant to and partner of McKinsey and Company in London. In the past decade he has written many articles about the problems of national health systems.

Christopher Robbins is Administrative Officer in the Social Affairs Division of the Council of Europe.

Aviva Ron, Sc.D., is Director of the Division of Planning and Information of the Kupat Holim Health Insurance Institution and Lecturer in Community Medicine at the Tel Aviv University Medical School.

Ernest W. Saward, M.D., is Professor of Social Medicine and Associate Dean for Extramural Affairs at the University of Rochester School of Medicine and Dentistry. Before taking up this position, he was Medical Director of the Kaiser Foundation Hospitals and Kaiser Foundation Health Plan in Portland, Oregon (1945–1970). Dr. Saward has served on the boards of numerous health organizations, and he has published widely in medical journals.